# The Asperger *Plus* Child

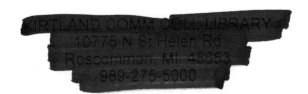

# The Asperger *Plus* Child

## How to Identify and Help Children with Asperger Syndrome and Seven Common Co-Existing Conditions*

*\*Bipolar Disorder, Nonverbal Learning Disability, Obsessive Compulsive Disorder, Oppositional Defiance Disorder, High-Functioning Autism, Tourette's Syndrome, and Attention Deficit Disorder*

George T. Lynn, M.A., M.P.A., L.M.H.C.
With Joanne Barrie Lynn

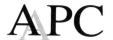

P.O. Box 23173
Shawnee Mission, Kansas 66283-0173
www.asperger.net

# APC

© 2007 Autism Asperger Publishing Co.
P.O. Box 23173
Shawnee Mission, Kansas 66283-0173
www.asperger.net

Publisher's Cataloging-in-Publication

Lynn, George T., 1945-

    The Asperger *plus* child : how to identify and help children with Asperger syndrome and seven common co-existing conditions (bipolar disorder, nonverbal learning disability, obsessive compulsive disorder, oppositional defiance disorder, high-functioning autism, Tourette's syndrome, and attention deficit disorder) / George T. Lynn ; with Joanne Barrie Lynn. -- 1st ed. -- Shawnee Mission, Kan. : Autism Asperger Pub. Co., 2007.

    p. ; cm.

    ISBN-13: 978-1-931282-33-8
    ISBN-10: 1-931282-33-1
    LCCN: 2006932792
    Includes bibliographical references and index.

    1. Asperger's syndrome in children. 2. Autism in children. 3. Syndromes in children. I. Lynn, Joanne Barrie. II. Title.

RJ506.A9 L96 2007
618.92/858832--dc22          0611

Designed in Stone Sans and Stone Serif.
Printed in the United States of America.

# Table of Contents

# Preface

approach the topic of differential diagnosis of children with Asperger Syndrome with excitement and humility. I am excited to share the lesson I have learned about working with this population as a psychotherapist: Every child is different and once you understand the difference, you are two thirds of the way to removing barriers to success for the child.

I am humble, because to write this book I needed to glean the wisdom of master teachers, psychiatrists and developmental psychologists. I am a mental health counselor, not a classroom teacher, doctor, or researcher. I tip my hat, especially to teachers of children with autism and Asperger Syndrome. I hope I have not misdescribed the job that you do. I have incredible admiration for your patience and creativity. I hope I have not been too clumsy in my understanding of your methods and assessment practices.

I have learned an enormous amount about autism from my editor, Dr. Jennifer Durocher, assistant director, UM-NSU CARD (Center for Autism & Related Disabilities). Dr. Durocher showed uncommon patience in her work with me on this project, making sure that the writing was properly supported by the research. She taught me to discern approaches and theories that might work in daily practice but were not substantiated by rigorous scientific testing.

I also thank my son, Gregory Barrie Lynn, himself a person diagnosed on the autistic spectrum, for the insights he has given me about what it is like to live as a neurological outsider. These have been very useful conversations for my professional development and I hope they have also been useful to him in being resourceful in his life.

I collaborated with Joanne Barrie Lynn in the writing of her story "I Have A Fork," which is the only visible evidence of her participation in this work. Her actual involvement in the book was extensive, however. Many of the ideas seen in the pages that follow were refined in creative consultation with her. As a poet and Greg's mother, she is able to do the intrapsychic detective work to discern what *really* moves children to do the things that they do.

Unseen in this work also are the lives, experience, and wisdom of hundreds of my young clients who range in age from 6 to 26. Everything I write is informed by their voices advising me to listen my way to the truth and watch my assumptions.

I hope that this book is useful to parents, teachers, and other professionals working with children and teens with Asperger Syndrome and related challenges. Let me know what you think. I heartily welcome email feedback to GeorgeLynn@ChildSpirit.com.

– George T. Lynn

Introduction

# The Genius of the Child with Asperger Syndrome

I n each of the following chapters, I will outline the conditions often seen with Asperger Syndrome (AS) or mistaken for it. I will describe identifying features of different neurotypes and detail the challenges and gifts of each. Finally, I will suggest strategies for helping AS children who show the presence of other conditions that often accompany AS.

The diagnostic trail I lay out concludes with the Character Map – a diagnostic list – the subject of Chapter Nine. By the time you get to this chapter, you will have a clearer idea of the strengths and challenges of the children who inhabit each of the neurotypes described. Throughout, it is important to remember that a child is more than the sum of his diagnoses. He is not a bundle of symptoms. He is an individual onto himself with a personality as unique as a fingerprint. In addition, a certain genius guides him.

I do not use the term "genius" to mean very superior IQ. I use this term the way the ancient Greeks and Romans used it, to denote the *guiding spirit* of the child. This is an aspect of the child's desire for being and accomplishment that is seen from a very, very young age. This book and the summary provided by the Character Map are ways to recognize the outlines of a child's genius in his challenges and gifts.

I begin Part I of this book with Chapter One, in which I describe my idea of what AS looks like as a stand-alone condition. Then I describe the look and feel of AS when it comes in combination with bipolar disorder (BD), nonverbal learning disorder (NLD), obsessive compulsive disorder (OCD), and oppositional defiant disorder (ODD).

In Part II, I detail how AS is different from three look-alike diagnoses: high-functioning autism (HFA), Tourette's syndrome (TS), and attention deficit disorder (ADD). In Chapter Nine, I summarize the material presented up until then in a Character Map. The Character Map is a tool for developing a more accurate understanding of the spirit, inner life, struggles, and strengths of the child. It does so in the format of a "yes" or "no" checklist derived from material described in the foregoing chapters.

All the children described in this book show the presence of an unconscious hope that their particular genius will be recognized and accepted. To help them accomplish this, caregivers, including teachers, must know enough about the child's neurological type to understand the impact of brain differences on behavior so as to work *with* the child instead of against him. Referring to the genius metaphor, such caregivers are able to move with the positive spirit of the child's genius, not against it. They are able to educate rather than dominate it.

In the classical paradigm, the genius, or muse, also has a dark side. Typically, he or she (the Romans termed the female genius the "juno") is so greedy to know the special interest, or accomplishment, that a person may become obsessional or isolated from others in the pursuit of the special knowledge. Children with AS are no exception to this rule – light does not exist without shadow. The fact is that the small bodies and immature intelligence of any attention-different child, including those with AS, may not be able to contain the egotistical enthusiasm of the genius and so tend to act as if everyone else in his life exists to help the genius reach its goals. Our task is to help this child see that progress in his special interest is furthered through his interdependence with others.

Mostly it is the shadow of AS, the "dark" aspects of personality, that brings these kids to me for counseling. It is the more serious co-existing conditions that often come with AS that move parents to consult a mental health counselor – the depression, anxiety, BD, ODD, and OCD that cause these kids and their parents the most grief. Some suggest that great potential for accomplishment does not exist without the presence of shadow features such as loneliness, perfectionism, obsessionality, mood problems, high anxiety, temper dyscontrol, and, sometimes, psychosis.

It takes time, patience, and good listening practice to begin getting an idea of the genius of the child with AS. Genius rarely shows itself straight out. It is more easily seen in the child's fears, special abilities, and challenges. In this regard, there are some common themes for the child with AS. As a preschooler, one child may take to disassembling machines while another will take to playing music; yet another will be fascinated with animals and their traits. These predilections may or may not show the presence of the genius of a computer scientist, composer, or visionary zoologist. Observing a child's "odd" behavior is part of the detective work. This takes time and a loving eye.

I am pleased to include a story, "I Have A Fork," written by author and poet Joanne Barrie Lynn. Our intention in providing this fictional narrative is to bring the human dimension to the book and soften its clinical focus. Joanne wrote the story to give an idea of how complex and interesting it is to be around children who are both mightily challenged and magnificently gifted. She makes the point that to help a child, you have to see things through his eyes. This takes psychological detective work.

There is detective work required because children cannot and do not tell you what is going on in their psyches. Though each of five children may show the presence of the same symptom, you will not be able to help any of them until you understand how each experiences the symptom and how it relates to the greater pattern of the child's personality and what he believes he needs to do to get through the day.

## Diagnostic Confusions Surrounding Children with Asperger Syndrome

The complexity of a child's issues must be understood if a child is to get the help he needs. There are certain diagnostic confusions that parents, teachers, and medical service providers need to resolve if they are going to do the right thing for children with AS. For example:

- *How can one tell the difference between the presence of a child's special interest in his obsessive pursuit of success at a particular video game (characteristic of AS) and the tendency for obsessive hyperfocus of a child with ADD, which may result in the same behavior?* Both children may become very distressed when we require them to stop playing the game but, as suggested in Chapter Eight, different remedial strategies are in order if we are to help the child.

- *Does a child who shows features of an extremely flat feeling tone fit the neurotype of the child with autism and his tendency for severe sensory aversion or social withdrawal?*[1] Or is this child demonstrating the lack of energy and lethargy that accompanies depression in children with AS or ADD?

- *Should a child who has motor and vocal tics be diagnosed with TS alone, or are there features that suggest the presence of AS along with TS?* This is an important distinction, because if a child has TS as a stand-alone condition, he does not demonstrate the same cognitive differences as the child with AS. In fact, he may have a neurotypical cognitive style. Therefore, the medication regime and social and educational accommodations that are needed to help kids with TS and AS are quite different.

- *Do the fits of anger of a child with a diagnosis of AS show the presence of the high anxiety and low frustration tolerance of AS or do they suggest the presence of rage, which is a signature of pediatric BD?* The treatment strategies needed to help children with BD are very different from those needed to treat an AS child with an anxiety disorder.

    If I believe a child suffers from manic-depression and that his rage is related to that condition, I immediately recommend that he be evaluated for a mood disorder by a physician for the purpose of possibly prescribing a mood stabilizer. If I believe a child is not experiencing rage but anger related to anxiety and high frustration, on the other hand, I suggest that he be enrolled in psychotherapy to teach him stress management skills and develop his sense of courage to cope with adversity in his life. In addition, I may suggest that he receive medical evaluation for prescription of anti-anxiety medication. (In Chapter Two, I discuss the brain chemistry of rage and how it is different from anger or meltdown.)

• *Are the obsessions and compulsions seen in the behavior of a child diagnosed with AS secondary to the AS or are they evidence of the presence of a stand-alone condition of OCD?* The characteristic rigidity and high anxiety that accompany change of routine for kids with AS look a lot like OCD, but different treatment, parenting, and educational strategies are indicated depending on the primary diagnosis.

These and other diagnostic predicaments cry out for clarification. In this regard, I am fortunate to be able to reference my clinical experience with hundreds of children diagnosed with attention differences as well as a growing body of literature on childhood psychiatric disorders.

*A caveat is required here. I am not a researcher. I am a practicing psychotherapist. Many of the interventions I suggest, as well as the theoretical underpinnings for these interventions, are based on my personal experience of the inner worlds of the children I work with and what seems to work for them – what seems to help them be more resourceful in their lives. I have been fortunate to have hundreds of these "good teachers" in my practice. I have done some structured client research of my own to define common patterns among my clients but I would not term this scientifically rigorous research. I endeavor to cite background research where such "hard" research exists, but the conclusions are my own.*

## The Importance of Understanding the Positive Intention of Negative Behavior

In order to help a child, I need to understand the child's experience from the inside. This requires that I listen closely to her, exploring her joy and suffering and the strategies she uses to meet her needs and realize her goals. If I can suspend my need to fix a child's problem and just listen from the heart, the positive intention of her distressing behavior will become clear. Once I have an understanding of that intention, I am able to create other ways for the child to realize her goals without the side effect of the disturbing or destructive behavior. Let us look at some examples.

- A child who has temper tantrums at school may be demonstrating an inability to read the nonverbal cues of others and so assumes the worst in every situation. Therefore, the positive intention of the temper displays is to telegraph to staff "I do not understand what anyone is saying to me and I need someone to help me understand and to help translate the way I communicate with others."

- A child who is combative and argumentative with all adults in his life may be trying to communicate: "I am unable to cope with unpredictable or unexpected events. Fighting and arguing is the only way I know to give myself a sense of control." Though the child may not understand the brain mechanics, he has learned that interpersonal encounter raises the level of dopamine in his brain with an accompanying increase in endorphin levels and, therefore, he welcomes a good argument. It makes him feel good, and improves his focus.

- A child who responds to stress by hitting himself or banging his head on his desk may be trying to say, "I am beside myself with so much stress that I do not even feel that I exist. Banging my head on my desk tells me 'I am!' every time I do it."[2]

These are just a few examples of negative behavior with a positive intent. In the pages that follow, I will attempt to show why children with AS and co-occurring conditions do the things that they do, what their logic is for their sometimes distressing behavior, so that we can help them get their needs met more directly.

## Challenges as Strengths

The challenges of the child with AS may be viewed as direct aspects of his strength. In terms of the structure of this book:

1.  His obsessive pursuit of his special interest helps him stay focused despite his AS-related tendency toward absent-mindedness.

2.  His high anxiety makes him pay very careful attention to things and, although he does not know it, may eventually equip him, as an adult, to be a valued specialist in some area in which it is very important to pay close attention to things.

If you consider success to involve helping the child be "happy" and "satisfied" in his life, these dynamics, these extremes of character, are true symptoms in the medical sense and will be treated as such. However, if you consider success to be the child's realization of his genius, even if this comes at the cost of ease and enjoyment of life, you become less antagonistic toward these "symptoms" and more willing to see how they fit in. The boy diagnosed with AS who wants to be a scientist when he grows up is obsessed with his special interest because there is "work to do" and it is important work. He is not necessarily happy. He is developing his genius. As you become more accepting of the "what is" in your child's personality, you become more creative in helping him.

### The Genius of Children with Asperger Syndrome

The gift of children with AS is their ability to visualize beauty in perfect form and construct systems based on that principle. These children are interested in the minutiae of how things work, and they are able to put white-hot focus on the function of something to make it work better.

World culture is in great crisis and new answers are needed. Some suggest that the presence of so many children with AS signals that help is on the way. Evolution teaches us that species change their structure to accommodate changes in the environment. For example, humans most likely developed the practice of walking upright because it made them better hunters. The presence of so many kids with the special gifts of Asperger Syndrome and autism may be such an accommodation. Though this may seem like a romantic and flawed way of looking at psychopathology, history teaches us that many important breakthrough thinkers over the centuries fit the AS neurotype. Perhaps the occurrence of cataclysmic changes such as the Greenhouse Effect cries out for the unusual creativity offered by the unusual perspectives of our children. At some point, very creative and unusual creativity is needed.

Dr. Temple Grandin takes another approach to the relationship of autism to the subjection of nature. She uses the term "abstractification" to describe the tendency of the non-autistic mind to "live in our thoughts surrounded by our ideas of things." Grandin says that the degradation of nature and destruction of the environment happen because of people living in and working in cubicles. She says, "This is what happens when humans cut the anchor and drift away from practical experience and especially the experience of nature and the world of animals."

She suggests that people with autism think like animals. They are not afflicted with the neurotypical disorder of cognitive dissonance, of seeing what a person expects to see. Because autistic people see things afresh, visually, and in great detail, they have a much needed ability to find creative solutions to problems that neurotypicals just cannot see.[3]

Features of AS and autism are seen in the lives of many scientific luminaries; the greatest, really. These include Einstein and Tesla (inventor of AC/DC current), who showed the poor social pragmatics, along with powerful visual skill, original thinking, and obsessive dedication to work at the expense of relationships, that mark that lives of many great scientists and inventors.

It is a style of thinking that needs to survive, not be pathologized. The first step is to recognize features of the pattern in our children. The second step is to come up with realistic ways to help them be "contenders," to help them realize their special gifts, and give us the benefit of their genius.

# Endnotes

1.  Prince-Hughes, D. (2004). *Songs of the gorilla nation: My journey through autism.* New York: Harmont Books; Williams, D. (1992). *Nobody nowhere – The extraordinary autobiography of an autistic.* New York: Avon Books.

2.  Williams, 1992. p. 211.

3.  Klinkenborg, V. (2005, May). What do animals think? (An interview with Dr. Temple Grandin). *Discover*, 46-52.

# Part I

Strategies for Helping Children with Asperger Syndrome Plus Bipolar Disorder, Nonverbal Learning Disability, Obsessive Compulsive Disorder, and Oppositional Defiance Disorder

Chapter One

# The Gifts and Core Challenges
# of Asperger Syndrome

**"I** was just like he is when I was a kid. I do not see what the big deal is. However, they are concerned about him at school, so I figured I would bring him here to get your opinion on why he acts the way he does and what I can do to help him. I think I would have liked someone to pay this kind of attention to me when I was his age."

I am a mental health therapist, and this is a statement I often hear from the fathers of the AS children I see in my practice. My office is located in the heart of the information technology-rich Seattle area, so I deal with many of the sons and daughters of folks employed in the computer field. Many of the fathers of my young clients show distinct features of AS, so it is no surprise that their children also demonstrate characteristics of this condition. In fact, this kind of "pass-along" is suggested by current research.[4]

I have learned from my interactions with this clientele that far from being a detriment to their life success, "having Asperger Syndrome" can be a huge success factor. Though AS parents may need help expressing their emotional sides, their genius working with ideas and machines has benefited them in their careers.

It does not seem to make sense to categorize Asperger Syndrome as a psychiatric illness when you look at the tremendous contributions people with AS have made to our culture. This is not to say that children with AS do not need a lot of help. Being born with a low emotional IQ, great difficulty behaving in socially appropriate ways, and a tendency to hyperfocus on their special interests are issues that require attention if they are to meet typical developmental milestones.

Although Asperger's Disorder is listed in the DSM-IV[5] (*Diagnostic and Statistical Manual*) as a psychiatric condition, people with AS do not suffer from "disordered thought" and do not have a "mental illness." They have a different way of thinking and solving problems. Dr. Lorna Wing, who wrote the diagnosis for Asperger Syndrome, stated:

> All the features that characterize Asperger Syndrome can be found in varying degrees in the normal population. People differ in their levels of skill in social interaction and in their ability to read nonverbal social cues. There is an equally wide distribution in motor skills. Many who are capable and independent as adults have special interests that they pursue with marked enthusiasm.[6]

It is important to note that Dr. Wing did detect comorbid psychiatric illness in the lives of many of the persons she included in her study, but she pointed out throughout her paper that the syndrome itself was not pathologic. This being said, there is no doubt that some, not all, persons with AS or high-functioning autism are impaired in terms of daily life functioning. Inasmuch as the central purpose of the DSM-IV is to define both psychological and developmental conditions that may be the focus of treatment, it is appropriate to include them.

Although children with AS features tend to behave in "odd" or unusual ways and often are friendless because of social skills deficits, they are not psychiatrically disturbed. They may need accommodations at school and they certainly need understanding and help from their parents and others to fit in, but these are essentially social conformity problems. There is no major pathology in their minds although they may process information in a unique way due to neurological differences.

My work with children diagnosed with AS has led me to believe that the AS child's drive to know all there is to know about something has a positive function for him. My perspective on this is shared by researchers such as Dr. Simon Baron-Cohen. The child with AS is successful *because* he is obsessional, rigid, pedantic, and lacks emotional range. These qualities equip him to succeed in areas that require a high degree of specialization and single-minded attention. They are perfect for him.[7]

## Asperger Syndrome as a Stand-Alone Condition

The patterns of giftedness and challenge seen in children with AS form a type of personality that is as characteristic of AS as the sunny, jovial, community-oriented type of personality is characteristic of Williams's syndrome and, to some degree, Down syndrome. Yet, the pattern is very unlike these two conditions. It is not jovial. It is typically intense, pedantic, dogged, obsessional, and joyful in accomplishment.

In the Introduction I noted that to be successful in my work of helping children with AS have better lives, I must get in touch with their genius, which I defined as their guiding spirit – an aspect that is both part of them and somewhat separate from them. The brilliant and iconoclastic manner of children with AS is the outward face of their genius. I have come to know and respect this muse and enjoy its company. I have also witnessed how this type of genius may cause others to suffer, particularly others who love the child. Raising a child with these features of character challenges the hardiness of even the hardiest parent and teacher. There are reasons why Hans Asperger included the term "malicious" in his description of the population.[8] Though not intentionally harmful, the lack of pragmatics and emotional clumsiness of children with AS may seem deliberately hurtful and, at times, malicious.

Our first task is to know and accept the child's genius. The second is to help him keep friends, loved ones, and important colleagues in his corner so that he may realize his dreams. We begin this process with a quick review of the DSM-IV diagnosis. In doing this, we do not endorse the idea that these symptoms show the child's "brokenness." They are indicators of how different his personality is from that of other kids. When he is an adult, he may be paid very well for manifesting each one of these symptoms at work; they will be tolerated for the greater good of the enterprise. However, as a child, these features of character sometimes make him so uncooperative that he is difficult to live with.

In order to properly track a child's needs and communicate with him, we must know the markers of his neurotype, and these markers are quite accurately described in the DSM-IV. In fact, all of the symptoms listed for Asperger's Disorder in the DSM-IV can be useful in different contexts.

## *An Overview of the Diagnosis of Asperger Syndrome*

In 1944, Dr. Hans Asperger, the head of the Department of Pediatrics at the University of Vienna, Austria, identified a population of his patients who showed interesting features of personality that would later be put together as a diagnosis. These included poor social skills, narrow repetitive behaviors, interests and routines, and the suggestion of antisocial and malicious behaviors. The children he wrote about had typically huge vocabularies with less understanding of what the words they said meant. They also had a pedantic and "little professor" way of communicating with people.

The DSM-IV diagnosis contains the following diagnostic criteria for Asperger's Disorder (299.80):

1. First there must be a qualitative impairment of "social interaction" as exemplified by the presence of at least two of items a. through d.:
   a. Impairment in the use of nonverbal behaviors such as eye contact, facial expression, body postures, and gestures to regulate social interactions
   b. Failure to develop appropriate developmental level
   c. Lack of spontaneous seeking to share enjoyments and interests
   d. Lack of social or emotional reciprocity

2. There must also be a "restricted patterns of behavior" present as indicated by the presence of at least one of items e. through h. below:
   e. Presence of a special interest that is abnormal in intensity and focus
   f. Inflexible adherence to nonfunctional routines or rituals
   g. Stereotypical and repetitive motor mannerisms (hand flapping, finger twisting)
   h. Preoccupation with parts of objects

3. And, there is no clinically significant general delay in language (e.g., single words used by age 2 years, communicative phrases used by age 3 years).

This last descriptor is written into the AS diagnosis in an attempt to differentiate it from autism. These differences, and the controversy over the contention that AS is simply a point on the autism continuum, a kind of high-functioning autism, will be discussed in detail in Chapter Six.

Both autism and Asperger's Disorders are included in the DSM-IV under a broad category referred to as Pervasive Developmental Disorders (PDD). This diagnostic category includes Autistic Disorder, Asperger's Disorder, and a catchall diagnosis called Pervasive Developmental Disorders-Not Otherwise Specified (PDD-NOS). This diagnosis is sometimes given by physicians and psychologists when the child exhibits characteristics similar to those seen in autism and AS, but does not meet the strict diagnostic criteria for either disorder.

Also included in the broad PDD category are two "degenerative" disorders involving significant loss of skills and functioning: Rett's disorder and Childhood Disintegrative disorder. Rett's disorder primarily affects girls and results in a loss of language and motor skills, including purposeful use of one's hands. Children with Childhood Disintegrative disorder exhibit a rapid and significant loss of social and communication skills, resulting in severe symptoms of autism. This "regression" occurs after a long period of normal development (typically between 3 and 10 years of age), and is different from the regression in language development and social interest that sometimes occurs between 18 and 30 months for children with autism.

## Parents' Reports of How Symptoms Emerge in Children with Asperger Syndrome

Asperger Syndrome is most challenging for children in the elementary school years. The good news is that the brain continues to grow and become more complex and more creative in terms of personal adaptation through adolescence. Toward the end of adolescence and into the twenties, the frontal lobes of the brain go through a final growth spurt. The frontal lobes of the left and right brain hemisphere are the seat of "executive function," and improvement in executive function is good news for the person with AS.

Executive function refers to a constellation of cognitive abilities that include the ability to plan, organize, and sequence tasks and manage multiple tasks simultaneously. My clinical observations and research[9] on the subject show that persons properly diagnosed with HFA have a more difficult time later in life with executive function. However, persons properly diagnosed with AS have an easier time accommodating to the demands of the neurotypical world for executive function although they still have difficulties that will be described later in this chapter.

Parents of children with AS report that social problems associated with the condition emerged early in their child's life. Around age 4, they report, the child fell out of step with the other kids. He started having temper tantrums. He had a difficult time understanding the motivations of other kids and was overly reactive. He might be identified by his preschool teacher as "overly aggressive." He needed everything to be predictable and could not function without structure.

As a preschooler, many parents relate, their child was very anxious around other children and preferred to play in parallel with children who were not threatening. The child did not understand the ordinary rules of social behavior and childhood games such as chase and "you've got it, I want it." He became upset and helpless when other children encountered him directly for play or in anger.

In elementary school, the child's socially awkward behavior caused him to experience problems on the playground. Whereas a neurotypical child knows better than to walk past a group of bullies who hang out on a certain part of the playground, a child with AS may blithely walk into their midst. The lack of common sense shown in doing so makes the child a target of the bullies and of other children who take advantage of his gullibility to talk him into perpetrating mischief while they make a quick getaway. Lacking common sense, the child with AS does not display sufficient guile to get away with the mischief and is easily caught.

Parents say that their AS child did not understand the meaning of the nonverbal behavior of the schoolyard bullies and did not understand what their smirking and whispering meant in this context. He could not read their nonverbal cues and therefore could not read their intentions. This is the meaning of the statement that he lacks the ability to "read others' minds."

It may be difficult for the neurotypical reader to understand this way of thinking because we (neurotypicals) instinctively "imagine" what others are thinking. Consider that the word "imagine" means "make an image of" or "picture in your mind," and you get an idea of what the child with AS cannot do. He cannot make the leap to accurate imagination or accurate assumption of what others are thinking, intending, or experiencing.

Many children with AS have great difficulty summoning the memory of their own experience as a way to understand another's verbal and nonverbal expressions of emotion and intention. The type of memory I am describing here is termed "implicit memory" to denote the fact that it is a type of "body/emotion" memory that is not evoked with the phrase "Oh yes, I remember ..." Rather, implicit memory is the type of memory that causes a person to react "out-of-consciousness" to any ordinary environmental event that, though not recalled in conscious memory, is encoded in an emotional reaction.[10]

If implicit memory is impaired, it is difficult for a person to react "intuitively" to his experience. Intuition, in this case, means the automatic cross-compare, analysis, and decision that occur without the mediation of conscious, logical decision-making. An example would be the physiological cues, or startle reactions, that are evoked instantaneously when we encounter a situation that is similar to a traumatic situation that was experienced in the past.

The AS child is challenged by difficulty understanding the meaning of anything that is described emotionally. He is very literal. "A is always A." This characteristic perceptual style makes it difficult for him to understand figures of speech – the essentially irrational constructions people use to convey the emotional flavor or intensity of some event. A figure of speech is a nonsense phrase that cuts right to the emotion without bothering with the facts. AS kids loathe figures of speech because they add a dimension of meaning to a description (emotion) that they, as children with Asperger Syndrome, cannot understand.

For example, the figure of speech "It's raining cats and dogs" is understood almost automatically by neurotypicals, who decode the emotional meaning as "It is raining so hard it is like dogs and cats were dropping from the sky on me. It was ferocious! And it was as if the dogs were chasing the cats. It was chaotically wet! It was an overwhelming rainstorm!" The child with AS has difficulty understanding this phrase because he cannot suspend his literal reality and imagine the emotional intensity of the event with all its layered emotional meanings and therefore understand the physical reality it describes.

Trying to communicate with an AS child using figures of speech or demanding an emotional response typically goes nowhere and may cause her to become angry or upset. The child may respond in frustration with the following statement: "What do you mean, 'You're tied up and can't talk?' You are not tied up. I see no rope tying you up!" Or, she may be insistent in asking, "What do you mean when you say you have a hunch? Show it to me." Or the child may begin yelling indignantly, "I did *not* go ballistic. I did not turn into a bullet! I have to know what you meant by that remark!"

Children diagnosed with AS are often described as lacking empathy – the ability to feel what others feel. This does not mean that they are callous toward others or want to hurt them. It means that they have difficulty with the neurological processes that allow them to categorize, remember, and cross-compare emotional information. This makes it difficult for them to quickly and flexibly generate appropriate emotional responses to situations affecting others. In fact, given the right situation, they may express considerable empathy. For example, a child with AS may show an empathetic emotional response in relating to others in his family or family pets because he has had sufficient *time* to observe and imprint the emotional reactions of these significant others.

## What Makes Asperger Syndrome Asperger Syndrome?

The essential difference between AS and every other diagnosis in this book is that children with AS have a very distinctive way of taking in everything around them. Specifically, they have a "fixed-figure" perceptual style. In order to explain this term, I need to digress for just a moment.

Perceptual psychologists suggest that people learn through a process of (a) focusing on individual objects or figures against their background; (b) taking in information about the object; and (c) letting the object recede back into general focus or background (the field). This happens very much the way a video camera lens highlights objects in the center of the scene against an indistinct background. Learning is accomplished in a sequence of focus on shifting "figures" in and out of the background.

The branch of psychology that is most interested in this process in terms of learning, development, and psychotherapy is Gestalt psychology. The terms "Gestalt" means field or background in German and the process of moving from one figural object to another is termed the "contact cycle."[11]

The pioneering developmental psychologist Jean Piaget said that the brain grows because of *assimilation* and *accommodation*. Going through the contact cycle, the child assimilates information about some new object and then accommodates to the new information by taking it into memory and making it part of his experience base.[12]

Making contact in this way is like breathing. Breathe in; breathe out; pause. The child concentrates on one figure. Something else attracts him. He goes to understand it. Breathe in; he takes it in. New ground forms around the figure. He takes it in deeper, now accommodating to it. Breathe out. Pause. If the rhythm is right, the child moves from one figure to the next all day long. Learning is natural, marked by development in intellectual and sensory capacity. Figure may be something in the environment. It may be some new emotional experience such as love or infatuation. It may be some new delight or some new terror. All experience shapes his neurological database, and as a result he is able to be more resourceful in his life, and his thought process becomes more complex.

The work of Dr. Uta Frith and other researchers, as well as my own observation of the children I work with, suggests that children with AS do not move easily around the Big Picture that contains all the "figures," all the points of interest, all the details, but get stuck on one aspect of the field. They have difficulty generalizing from one experience to another, from one piece of knowledge to another, or from one emotional event to another. They do not have the ability to move from one object of focus to another in a fluid, flexible way.

I have learned in over 15 years of working with kids with AS that they do not see the forest through the trees. Although they may be very well versed in their special interest, they tend to have difficulty with open-ended creativity. True to Dr. Wing's diagnosis, they tend to get fixated on the details of any aspect of inquiry and may become agitated if asked to take a wider perspective on the issue. In fact, they are often ignorant of the context, fail to "get the point," or "understand the central theme" that pulls details together.

Here are some examples of the AS tendency toward fixed-figure perception.

---

**Examples of Fixed-Figure Perception in Children with AS**

- Can only focus on one thing at a time and become very upset if pulled off focus.

- Argue miniscule facts of a situation ad infinitum.

- Lack the ability to see the Big Picture with regard to their own behavior, or in general, and have a difficult time seeing others' perspectives in problem solving.

- Do not understand the shared emotional wisdom of jokes and stories.

- Go very deep into a subject but do not cross-compare with other topics unless directed to do so.

- Are called by others "the ultimate nit picker" or "typical left-brained engineer type."

- Are vocationally drawn to technology and are technically creative – brilliant in answering closed-category questions about their field.

---

Dr. Uta Frith has suggested that the term "lack of central coherence" or "weak central coherence"[13] describes the behavior of children with AS and autism that I term the "fixed-figure" perceptual style.

With due respect for her work, I am not using Frith's term to describe children with AS because I believe that their perceptual process is not the same as that of children with HFA. Children with AS do demonstrate (in Frith's terms) impaired ability to have a "coherent," meaningful understanding of their experience and how things relate together. But, in my experience, the child with HFA is better described as experiencing a condition I have labeled "full-field" perception; that is, she is cognitively blasted by all stimuli coming at her at once and experiences great difficulty separating objects of focus from each other. Unlike the AS child stuck in focus on one special tree, the HFA child is stuck in a wide-open focus on the whole forest, unable to zoom in to learn about individual trees.

Children with AS have a powerful advantage over children with HFA in that they can use language to create categories for their interests and thus remember important facts. They can use language to put things in order in their minds: "I put this piece here. It is my special interest. I bridge from it to look at that piece. Now I look at that piece and ask myself what relationship does it have to my special interest?"

Some readers may counter my assertion that children with HFA do not show a lack of central coherence by pointing out that a part of the diagnosis for both AS and HFA is the language around "preoccupation with parts of objects." I would respond that although children with HFA show fascination with the tiny details of things (Dr. Frith talks about how they might "zoom in on the pattern of a decorated china tea cup"), there is an essential difference in the function that this interest in details plays for them. As I will argue in Chapter Six, children with HFA tend to focus on the details of things or have special interests as a *reaction* to a sense of being *overwhelmed* by stimulation around them. In children with AS, however, the cause of this kind of selective focus is more likely a compensation for the inability to see the Big Picture in the first place. This brings us to examine how preference for fixed-figure or immobile full-field perception develops.

### When Do Children "Develop" AS or HFA?

My interviews with parents of my AS and HFA clients reveal that many of these children seemed to be very much alike until around the age of 2. But something happened between 15 and 30 months of age. It was if the child's neurology turned and he started showing features of AS (fixed-figure preference) or HFA (immobile full-field preference).

One study found that at some point in early childhood development, children may become brain specialized either on the left or the right side of the cortex. If a child becomes specialized to the left side, he develops AS.[14] If he becomes specialized to the right side, he becomes autistic. I describe the impact of right-hemisphere specialization in Chapter Six. Below I touch on the impact of left-hemisphere specialization for children with AS.

The price that children with AS pay for becoming specialized to the left side of their brains is that they have a very difficult time getting outside their own limited interests and views to see things differently or see others' perspectives. They remain, in Jean Piaget's term, very "egocentric." And, borrowing another term from Piaget, they have severe problems with "centration;" that is, they have a powerful tendency to focus only on one aspect of any object of interest.

Part of the issue may be that not having full access to the right hemisphere of the brain, they do not have full use of the orbitofrontal cortex (OFC), a structure located in the frontal cortex of the brain, bilaterally over the eyes. The OFC is responsible for providing awareness of background and context so that people can make meaning from their experience. The right-side orbitofrontal cortex is involved in this kind of meaning-making, and underfunction of this part of the structure may be part of the problem children with AS have keeping things in a larger perspective.[15]

Their loss of right-brain ability is revealed in their difficulty with a variety of tasks that involve this cerebral hemisphere. Specifically, children with AS are impaired in the ability to:

- Do more than one thing at a time or take more than one piece of information in at a time.

- Accurately judge where their bodies are in space – they tend to be clumsy; their nervous systems do not do a good job of cross-comparing and integrating the thousands of miniscule small movements and impulses that make up large movements.

- Have flexible movements in facial muscles and use gestures to express themselves nonverbally.
- Cross-compare information between domains that are not directly connected (open-ended creative thought).

Within their specialty people with AS can be very creative. If they are focusing on a system, they can make the system work much better. People with AS go *deep* into one thing and make their contribution there, but they do not go *wide*. Depending on their area of interest, they may or may not achieve breakthrough success in their chosen areas of science and technology.

### How to Assess a Child's Perceptual Style as Showing Fixed-Figure or Full-Field Perception

In order to influence a child, to teach him and parent him, you have to know his perceptual style and his limitations in that regard. Children with HFA, for example, have a very difficult time understanding how to break problems into manageable pieces and are unable to follow written instructions. Children with AS may find it almost impossible to understand the concept of interdependence embodied in the Golden Rule. They are too egocentric.

It is important to know these facts about a child if you are going to achieve rapport with her – if you are going to get through to her and help her develop compensation strategies:

1.  Ask the child to describe some recent event that has occurred in her life from beginning to end, such as a hike or a birthday party.

    Many HFA children are not able to do this because, though they may have an image of the event, they are not able to "deconstruct" the memory into its separate sequential parts and describe it to you. Unlike the child with HFA, the child with AS is typically able to give you an extremely detailed account of the event down to tiny details once she gets started with the process.

2.  Give the child a jumble of parts with a picture of the finished project and see how quickly she can assemble some structure from the parts.

    You can use any kind of building set that has snap-together parts, such as Legos or Knex. Typically, children with HFA move quickly on this type of project because they are able to use their well-developed visual skills to imagine the result and then build to this result. Children with AS tend to nit-pick the details and have a hard time putting it all together: It just has to be perfect before they will move to the next step.

3.  Verbally give the child a problem and see how she goes about solving it. A child with HFA may simply sit there without reacting, unable to begin the process of deconstructing what you have said. She understands that you want her to do something but cannot make heads or tails of your description of the problem. As Dr. Temple Grandin and others have suggested, people with autism think in pictures, and if a complex symbolic, analytic task is before them, it may take them a long time to come up with valid conclusions because they solve problems by comparing pictures, whole Gestalts, and relying on their intuitive skills to generate new pictures, new possibilities for the problem situation.

    A child with AS, on the other hand, will give you an immediate response and may be very verbal. In fact, she may be perseverant, obsessive, highly anxious, and robotic-looking, but she is *engaged* in the struggle for understanding and success.

## *Heritability Factors for Asperger Syndrome*

Results from twin studies indicate that if one identical twin is diagnosed with AS, there is a 90% chance his twin will also meet the diagnostic criteria for AS.[16]

In my clinical practice, I have never come across a child who truly fit the AS neurotype who did not have a close relative with the diagnosis or who showed the essential features of AS in his or her life. Though I would not make the diagnosis *because* a child has a first-degree relative with AS, if I do not find such an ancestor, I am more cautious in making a diagnosis of AS.

Most frequently it is a child's father, grandfather, or uncle who most closely fits the AS diagnosis. Males with AS outnumber females three to one in the identified population.[17] Occasionally the behavior, interests, and affective style of female relatives show presence of AS. If both parents fit the AS diagnosis, there is a high probability that one or more of their children also do. I look for signs of the presence of AS in my initial intake with parents, including the following: What are the child's parents' professions? Typically, at least one of the parents works in a scientific or technical field.[18]

A recent study of 1,000 families found that fathers and grandfathers (patri- and matrilineal) of children with autism or AS were more than twice as likely to work in the field of engineering compared to control groups. Indeed, 28.4% of children with autism or AS had at least one relative (father and/or grandfather) who was an engineer. Related evidence comes from a survey of students at Cambridge University conducted by Baron-Cohen studying either sciences (physics, engineering, or math) or humanities (English or French literature). When asked about family history of a range of psychiatric conditions (schizophrenia, anorexia, autism, Down syndrome, language delay, or manic depression), the students in the science group showed a six-fold increase in the rate of autism in their families, and this was specific to autism.

***Predictable AS family success patterns.*** Who are the characters in the family genogram? (A genogram is a family tree diagram that represents the names, birth order, sex, and relationships of the members of a family.) And what were their accomplishments? I find many noted scientists, innovators, inventors, and people who just loved tinkering with machines. These people were decidedly more interested in the relationships between objects and ideas than they were in the relationships between people.

## Common Myths About Asperger Syndrome

Contrary to popular opinion, people with AS may appear typical and be able to practice neurotypical-looking social skills and be quite "normal" in other ways, including the following:

- *Eye contact and a sense of humor.* Though children with AS find it difficult to make eye contact, many AS adults have learned to relax their gaze or look at the space between the listener's eyes and right over the nose.

- *Graceful movement when practiced.* As I note in *Survival Strategies for Parenting Children with Bipolar,*[19] quite a few of the AS kids I have worked with are noted for their expertise in a martial art. They do not develop excellence because of inborn grace and intuition but because of grueling, constant, daily practice.

- *Sexual desire.* My observation from my work with adolescents with AS is that the level of sexual desire (ongoing interest in sex) is somewhat less than that of the neurotypical population. These kids voice a lot of confusion with regard to personal sexual identity as well as mores and taboos around sex. They are typically woefully uninformed about appropriate behavior in this domain. In younger AS children, gender identity problems may be present but these issues usually fade by late adolescence.[20]

- *Creative ability.* Creativity is found in the area of the child's special interest, especially in putting discrete facts together to form a conclusion or solve a design problem. This type of creativity is quite different from the "what if" creativity, the ability to brainstorm different scenarios, that is seen in the neurotypical population.

# Conclusion: See Asperger Syndrome as a Way of Thinking, Not a Pathological Condition

The title of this chapter suggests that there are specific gifts, a specific genius, that come with AS. This may eventually give the child a powerful one-up in the information age. On one occasion, one of my adult AS clients shared that when he was in high school he was a social pariah, friendless, and lonely. He used to passionately envy the popular boys who seemed to have everything going their way. A couple of these neurotypical kids permitted him to hang around them but never invited him to parties or took him seriously. Now, my client reported, these boys, grown to men, deliver bottled water to his office on the 14th-floor corner suite of a new building in Redmond near Microsoft headquarters. The social skills that served the popular boys so well in high school could not compete with the focused brilliance of my client in pursuit of his special interests – science, technology, and computers.

Given the right accommodations, children with AS have a good chance of meeting typical developmental milestones (though they may do so several years after neurotypicals), have good careers, and eventually find others with whom to share their lives.

It is important to point out that some research[21] suggests that many people with AS do not achieve economic independence and remain "worthy dependents" into adulthood. For this reason, I am cautious when I discuss the probable futures of children with AS with these kids' parents. I do not want to give the false impression that all AS children become successful and that if a child does not reach her goals, it is somehow her parents' fault. Typically, the problem is more the child's brain chemistry and structure than any deficit in the care provided by parents.

As a therapist, I must avoid "flight into futility" predilection that vexes other professionals who do not have to provide both a realistic and a positive vision of the possibilities of children with neuropsyche issues. I focus on the positive because my instinct, honed by working for more than 25 years in the counseling field, is that people do not change simply because you tell them what is "wrong" with them. They have to pull toward strength.

With regard to the pessimistic research data, I suggest it is important to consider that many of the studies lump kids with HFA and AS together – the commonly held belief is that both conditions are "on the spectrum" of autism. Given the potentially profound developmental delays of people with autism, putting these two diagnoses together may drag down the curve unrealistically for people with AS. In addition, there is a greater chance that people will end up in research studies if they have more extreme aspects of AS or HFA or more co-morbidities. The people who inhabit the executive suites at Microsoft are not written about in these studies because they have gotten through without being marginalized.

Repeating a theme first stated in the Introduction, the genius of children with AS may be seen in the intersection of two lines of innate talent. First, all these children have the ability to apply white-hot *focus* to their special interests. They do not give up in the pursuit of knowledge and skill about this interest. They learn it well and so completely that they are capable of breakthrough thinking and innovation. In addition, I believe, along with Dr. Simon Baron-Cohen, that they share another major feature of the genius of children on the autistic spectrum: They are driven to understand *systems* – the way in which natural or man-made phenomena interact toward a goal.[22]

The interest in systems is one of the reasons why AS children warm up so readily to computers. In this technology, they find both an algorithm for human intelligence (without emotions) and perfectly interacting processes that (in systems terms) proceed from designated inputs to outputs. Many children with AS are fascinated by system function to include mechanical devices such as automobiles, medicine, or medical technology, and natural systems such as animal species, rivers, or cosmic phenomena. They are eager to find out how things fit together and how natural and human-made systems interrelate. Dr. Temple Grandin speaks for many on the autism spectrum when she states, "I am deeply interested in the new chaos theory, because it means that order can arise out of disorder and randomness. I've read many popular articles about it, because I want scientific proof that the universe is orderly."[23]

---

### The Positive Genius of Asperger Syndrome

- Ability for white-hot focus on the special interest.

- A craving to understand how systems work and a delight in improving their function.

- Searching for perfect patterns in target of interest. Observes important details that make the difference and goes deep enough to find answers others cannot see.

---

So we begin the exploration of this interesting and culturally needed neurotype with the observation that there is perfection in the character of children with the AS diagnosis. And, using the model of the Genius in the Bottle, the power of the child's personality must be understood and contained if she is to grow to successful adulthood.

The job of parents and teachers of children with AS is to get the child to the second stage of life, adulthood, in one piece. Once there, the predilection for specialized thinking can become an asset. In the chapters that follow we attempt to contribute to caregivers' success in this endeavor by discussing what AS looks in combination with other conditions; what it is and what it is not.

## Endnotes

4. Muhle, R., Trentacoste, S. V., & Rapin, I. (2004). The genetics of autism. *Pediatrics, 113*(5), 72-86; Bailey, A., Lecouteur, A., Gottesman, I., Bolton, P., & Simonoff, E. (1995). Autism as a genetic disorder: Evidence from a British twin study. *Psychological Medicine, 25*, 63-77; Gilberg, C. (1989). The borderland of autism and Rhett Syndrome: Five case histories to highlight diagnostic difficulties. *Journal of Autism and Development Disorder, 19*, 545-559.

5. American Psychiatric Association. (2000). *Diagnostic and statistical manual of mental disorders* (4th ed.; text revision). Washington, DC: Author.

6. Wing, L. (1981). Asperger Syndrome: A clinical account. *Psychological Medicine, 11*, 115-129.

7. Baron-Cohen, S. (2000, January). Is Asperger Syndrome/high-functioning autism necessarily a disability? [Invited submission for special millennium issue of *Development and Psychopathology* draft] *Cambridge University Press, 12*, 269-290.

8. Mesibov, G. (2000, November-December). High-functioning autism or Asperger Syndrome: Why the controversy? *Autism and Asperger's Digest,* 16-18.

9. Rinehart, N. J., Bradshaw, J. L., Brereton, A. V., & Tonge, B. J. (2002). Lateralization in individuals with high-functioning autism and Asperger's disorder: A frontostriatal model. *Journal of Autism and Developmental Disorders, 32*(4), 321-331.

10. Losh, M., & Capps, L. (2003, June). Narrative ability in high-functioning children with autism or Asperger Syndrome. *Journal of Autism and Developmental Disorders, 3*, 239-251.

11. Zinker, J. (1978). *The creative process in gestalt therapy.* New York: Vintage.

12. Piaget, J. (1972). *To understand is to invent.* New York: The Viking Press, Inc.

13. Fletcher, P., Happé, F., Frith, U., Baker, S., Dolan, R., Frackowiak, R., & Frith, C. D. (1995). Other minds in the brain: A functional imaging study of theory of mind in story comprehension. *Cognition, 57*(2), 109-128.

14. Rinehart et al., 2002.

15.  Sabbagh, M. (2004, June). Understanding orbitofrontal contributions to theory-of-mind reasoning: Implications for autism. *Brain and Cognition, 55*(1), 209-215.
16.  Bailey et al., 1995; Gilberg, 1989.
17.  Wing, L. (1993). The definition and prevalence of autism: A review. *European Child and Adolescent Psychiatry, 2,* 1-14.
18.  Baron-Cohen, 2000, January.
19.  Lynn, G. (2000). *Survival strategies for parenting children with bipolar disorder.* London, UK: Jessica Kingsley Publishers.
20.  Reiner, W. G. (2003). Normal and abnormal psychosocial development in children and adolescents. In *Recent breakthroughs in child and adolescent psychiatry.* Irvine, CA: CME, Inc. pp. 13-39.
21.  Howlin, P., Goode, S., Hutton, J., & Rutter, M. (2004). Adult outcomes in children with autism. *Journal of Child Psychology and Psychiatry, 45*(2), 212-229.
22.  Baron-Cohen, S. (2000, January).
23.  Grandin, T. (1995). *Thinking in pictures and other reports from my life with autism.* New York: Doubleday. p. 192.

Chapter Two

# Fire and Ice: Helping Children Cope with Asperger Syndrome Plus Bipolar Disorder

S ome of the most troubled children that I work with show signs of
having the dual challenges of Asperger Syndrome and bipolar disorder (BD). The lack of common sense that comes with AS and the
aggressive depression of bipolar illness in combination create enormous
challenges for the child and his parents.

This chapter describes the characteristics of children with early-
onset BD and suggests strategies to help children who experience a co-occurring AS plus BD. Treating a child with BD with appropriate medication
is the first order of business. Therefore, if I see evidence of this condition,
I immediately refer parents to a physician. At the same time, I work with
the parents and the child to construct strategies to deal with issues related
to the combined diagnosis.

Many parents come to me convinced that their child is "bipolar" because of severe temper tantrums, oppositionality, and problems at
school. I caution parents about jumping to the conclusion that their child
has BD without sufficient evaluation. I proceed carefully because this diagnosis is associated with the highest suicide rate of any listed in the DSM-IV.
Thus, misjudgment of clinical factors in dealing with this population can
have lethal consequences. If a child has co-existing AS, which limits his

ability to be practical or to reason his way through personal problems, the situation is grave indeed.

There is another reason why I proceed carefully when considering the possibility that a child has BD. That is because getting this diagnostic label radically changes the way the world looks at the child and the way he looks at himself. A key requirement for emotional development is that the child possess a positive autobiography – a sense of himself as worthy and powerful. There is a great deal of cultural misconception about BD, and these wrong-headed ideas may influence the child's caregivers to give him the wrong idea about himself. Although a misperception, BD is still some-times equated with psychopathology or antisocial personality disorder. For example, because one must take a mood-stabilizing drug, having the diagnosis precludes admittance to the U.S. Armed Forces. And the popular press often cites presence of this diagnosis when profiling famous villains such as the Seattle teacher, Mary Kay Latourneau, who was convicted of child rape.[24]

However, children and adults with BD are not sociopaths, serial killers, or criminals. They are people who are greatly challenged to control their emotional lives. And they are suffering.

Working with physicians who diagnose mood disorders in children has acquainted me with some alternative diagnoses that support the use of anticonvulsant medication (the type used to treat BD) to treat children with bipolar-like symptoms without labeling them with BD. These include "encephalopathy not otherwise specified (NOS)" – translation, "something is wrong with the brain;" or "cyclothymic disorder," which describes a mood-shift syndrome with less severe levels of symptoms than BD.

In Chapter One, I provided a description of Asperger Syndrome as a stand-alone condition to make clear the definitional aspects of the AS pattern. I move now to a description of pediatric BD as a way to develop an understanding of what BD adds to the personality of the child also di-agnosed with AS.

# Four Essential Markers of Child-Onset Bipolar Disorder

In my book *Survival Strategies for Parenting Children with Bipolar Disorder,*[25] I provide a 14-item checklist for evaluating the presence of BD in children. I will here refine this list to the top four qualities. In my interview with children and their parents, I take a careful inventory of these four factors, trying to determine the child's behavior and feeling states at home and school. If a child's affect, behavior, and thought processes meet the description of persons who experience BD on these four factors, I will refer for medical evaluation.

---

### Four Essential Markers of Child-Onset Bipolar Disorder

1. The presence of mood shift from mania or hypomania to depression or the "ultra-rapid cycling" mixed state.

2. The presence of manic-depression in the child's family tree.

3. The presence of psychosis and/or disordered thought.

4. The presence of rage as distinctly different from meltdown.

---

## *Evidence of Cycling Mood Shift from Mania or Hypomania to Depression?*

Bipolar disorder is defined by the existence of severe, cyclical shifts in mood between depression and mania. Depression is a state of extreme sadness, lethargy, and physical debilitation. It is as much a physical syndrome as a mental condition. When depressed, a person's respiration decreases. He fatigues easily and experiences pain and increased vulnerability to stress. Further, he loses (or greatly gains) appetite and experiences the inability to sleep or the inability to stay awake. He may also voice suicidal ideation. These features of depression, when seen in BD in children and adults, are more severe than when depression exists as a stand-alone condition.[26]

Dr. Hagop Akiskal, a leading authority on BD in children, suggests that the poor sleep habits these children experience (up all night, asleep during the day) and depression give them the appearance of a state he terms "hypersomniac retardation."[27]

Mania is defined as "inappropriately elevated expansive or irritable mood" when seen in adults. A manic person may be filled with fantastic and unrealistic optimism. He may believe that he will buy up all the real estate in the world and give it to the poor; perfect a time machine if only given a research grant to do so; or believe that he is capable of feats of extraordinary ability, such as walking across a busy freeway without getting hurt. The sky is the limit.

Research suggests that preadolescent children do not exhibit the "elevated and expansive mood" characteristic of adult-onset bipolar disorder. They will, however, demonstrate presence of rage, which may be a juvenile variation of the extreme irritability characteristic of mania.

Hypomania is the term used to describe less severe mania that does not disable the person in terms of everyday function. It will be seen in the child's very unrealistic expectations about his ability to achieve things in his life or in a hyper-energized creativity, a rush of ideas and pressured speech, that often occurs at nighttime.[28]

Mania may also be evidenced by a giddy, out-of-it appearance the child takes on. He may grimace and seem absent from his own mind. He goes about hyperactively annoying people or behaving in a generally dysinhibited manner. This is a state of consciousness one of the parents I work with terms "gibbon boy," to denote the "monkey-like" appearance of her hypomanic child.

Some children become dangerously impulsive. They may jump out of a moving car, climb up on the roof and dance, or ceaselessly torment every other person in the family, throwing things out of the refrigerator and toppling over furniture.

Bipolar disorder in children may come in the form of the so-called "ultra-rapid cycling" variety, which is seen in a shift from a depressed, possibly rageful, state to a manic or hypomanic state several times a day. Young children are more apt to experience drastic mood shift of the ultra-rapid cycling variety, and their depressive affect is most often expressed as fits of *rage* (see below for discussion of the rage reaction).[29]

Dr. Demitri Papolos, author of *The Bipolar Child: The Definitive and Reassuring Guide to Childhood's Most Misunderstood Disorder*, believes that BD in children and adolescents may be expressed in either extreme emotional "fight" or "flight" behavior. Of the adolescent clients I treat in my counseling practice, somewhat more girls fit the "flight" profile. They are prone to depressive collapse and are highly anxious. They are less impulsive and may express their hypomanic states in less destructive ways than kids who fit the "fight" profile in BD. They stay up all night writing or doing other creative work but they are not out carousing. Their circadian rhythm is much disrupted, and they tend to sleep during the day and be prone to school avoidance. They spend 80% of their time in a mild to serious depressive state and 20% in hypomania. Self-destructive impulsivity may lead to self-harming (such as cutting oneself) or suicidal behavior in these kids.[30]

If an adolescent is given more to the "fight" pattern of BD, he or she will have a different range of problems. Both mania and hypomania show up in these adolescents as destructive impulsivity such as law breaking, drug abuse, or sexual promiscuity. An adolescent in the active, aggressive, "fight" pattern of BD may go without sleep for days at a time. He may stay up at night buying things on the Internet with his parents' credit cards, or may be given to petty thievery and shoplifting.

All cycling mood conditions are not manic depression. Many children experience mood cycling from a normal, "euthymic" (good mood) to a depressed mood. Fluctuations (or "cycles") between normal and depressed or sad moods are common in adolescence and do not usually carry the severe challenges that accompany the presence of mania.

## The Look and Feel of Mania and Hypomania in Children, Teens, and Adults

| Feature | Child | Adolescent | Adult |
|---|---|---|---|
| Elevated mood/ mood shift | • Acts mindless and "monkey-like." <br> • Believes he has magical powers. <br> • Becomes unusually helpful to parents. | • Extremely happy, sociable, feels smarter, better than peers. <br> • Takes on too heavy of an academic load. <br> • Suddenly tearful. | • Feels "golden, on top of the world." <br> • Much increased goal-directed activity. <br> • Foolish decisions. |
| Rate of speech | Rapid, incessant. | Rapid, non-stop, very distractible. | Rapid, non-stop; cannot get a word in. |
| Sleep habits | • Difficulty going to bed or getting to sleep. <br> • Has night terrors. | Stays up all night on the Internet. Activates at night. | May miss several days of sleep, activates at night. |
| Racing thoughts | Cannot focus. Mind full of "great ideas." | • Difficulty listening or sitting still. <br> • Impatient. <br> • Suddenly creative. | Feels extremely creative all of a sudden. |
| Impulsivity | • Persistently intrusive. <br> • Does not wait turn. <br> • Poor frustration tolerance. | • Rule and law breaking. <br> • Dangerous sexual behavior. <br> • Poor frustration tolerance. | Rash judgments and self-destructive decisions. |

## Evidence of BD in Child's First-Degree Relatives?

There is abundant evidence from research of the family lines of children with BD to suggest that the condition has a genetic component.[31] If one parent is diagnosed with BD, there is at least a 40% probability that a child born of the couple will meet the diagnostic criteria for the disorder. If both parents show features of BD, there is a better than 60% probability that it will be passed on to children. Interesting, this research indicates that if a child is diagnosed with early-onset BD (by age 7) of the ultra-rapid cycling variety, there is a higher probability that the condition will be found in the child's maternal family line.[32]

When I do an assessment for BD in a child, I always query parents for information about the presence of manic depression in mother, father, grandparents, aunts, or uncles. In addition, because the exact diagnoses of first-degree relatives may not be clear, I ask about psychiatric hospitalizations, suicides, depression, and alcoholism. The presence of these life events in a child's family of origin is a clue to the presence of BD.

When gathering a child's family history, it is often difficult to identify if schizophrenia was part of the picture for any of his ancestors. In 1921, a German psychiatrist, Dr. Emil Kraepelin, identified a specific type of mental illness he called "manic-depression" that he separated from the illness that had previously been identified as schizophrenia. Despite his early identification of manic-depression, clinicians continued to misdiagnose it as schizophrenia until the early 1960s.[33]

There is a powerful degree of apparent similarity between the two conditions. Both may show extreme depressed affect, both may evidence psychosis, and both may show variations of mania. However, there are also remarkably profound differences. The primary features of schizophrenia – delusions, hallucinations, and paranoid behavior – tend to be more chronic. These phenomena do not come and go at predictable intervals, as does mood shift in BD. In schizophrenia there is a true loss of self; the person lives in a fantasy world and does not come out of this state of consciousness while the disease is running its course. Schizophrenia may result in the loss of intelligence. It is by far the worst, most profound, most disabling condition.

Bipolar disorder, on the other hand, is very treatable. By definition, symptoms emerge and fade. Dr. Demitri Papolos and other authorities on the disorder have pointed out that given appropriate medical treatment, people with BD have the chance of living truly splendid and successful lives.[34]

Though research indicates that BD is as frequently seen in persons with cognitive and developmental disabilities as in the nondisabled population, my clinical experience and contact with parents consistently point to the likelihood that high creativity and drive are part and parcel of the condition and will express the genius of the individual if managed with awareness, skill, and compassion for self.

## Symptoms of Psychosis?

Psychosis is diagnosed by the presence of auditory or visual hallucinations, severely distorted or disordered thought process, or "magical" thinking. About half of the children I work with who are diagnosed with BD experience visual hallucinations. For example, they see things that are not present in objective reality, such as people coming up the walk to their house or entities coming out of the wall. Though auditory hallucinations are less frequent, many children with the BD diagnosis tell me that they hear their names being called when they are by themselves.[35] Some children hear voices in their minds that express separate personalities.

Auditory and visual hallucinations may be quite benign (aside from the distress they cause the child simply due to their presence) or they may contain commands to do inappropriate or dangerous things or negative self-evaluations. Auditory or visual hallucinations that attack a child's self-esteem or contain commands to do something destructive to others are classified as dangerous hallucinations and should receive high priority for treatment.

Psychosis is also seen in "magical thinking" long past the time when a child should understand that he is not capable of performing magical feats such as hitting a baseball over a skyscraper or flying when he jumps off the roof of his house. The line between frank psychosis and mania is thin. The excitement a manic child feels as he climbs to the roof is part of the psychotic belief that he will not hurt himself in the process.

Disordered thought process may show itself as a mild paranoia – the child is unable to acknowledge his part in a situation even when confronted straight on with the evidence of his involvement. Disordered thought may also manifest itself in the child's inability to make sense of his own thoughts. He will articulate gibberish or "word salad." This troubling lack of control has been identified by research that shows that children who experience thought disorder could not put words and thoughts into their proper sequence in their minds or assign a priority to what they say.[36] Instead of speaking in logical, sequential form, thoughts will appear as if from nowhere and disappear just as fast. They may make sense for a few moments, then trail off into the abyss.

## *Rage or Meltdown?*

The experience of rage among children and teens with bipolar challenges is the most often cited reason why parents bring their children to my psychotherapy practice. Many psychotherapists see rage as the acting out or re-enactment of trauma. Rage may be related to child abuse, but this is not the only cause. By and large, the rage experienced by the children I work with is related to their particular genetic susceptibility to manic-depression. It is not a result of family dysfunction.

Meltdown is a different phenomenon. It is the "flight" aspect of the "fight or flight" reaction and, as such, does not indicate the presence of BD in a child's personality. To help the reader make this important distinction, I will profile the look and feel of rage in a child, then compare and contrast rage with meltdown.

***Rage.*** Rage is the take-over of the frontal cortex or thinking brain by the emotional brain – the limbic system.[37] The frontal cortex is usually successful at holding the "animal" energy of the limbic brain in check. But during rage, the limbic system takes over, flooding the cortex with impulses. As the cortex shuts down, the limbic brain consolidates its victory over the body. The screaming-laughing-crying and frothing-at-the-mouth of the enraged bipolar child is a dramatic expression of the limbic brain's power, and it is scary!

One child diagnosed with BD told me that the onset of rage surprised him. It was as if he were in a dark hallway being pursued by an ax murderer. He could let the menace have his body and mind (and express the rage) or he could jump into a "fiery pit" at the end of the hallway. The fiery pit was a metaphor for the feelings of extreme anger and annoyance at others that he would experience while he was inhibiting rage.

In BD, rage results from the collision of the manic and depressed phases of the disorder in the "mixed state" diagnosis. "Mixed state" is the term used to identify a person's mood when mania and depression occur simultaneously. Rage in children expresses the pitiless energy of bipolar depression with manic force. It is the epitome of the mixed state in children who do not have the coping skills to get their bodies under control and therefore become victim to the emotional storm noted by Dr. Hagop Akiskal.[38]

In this situation, rage expresses the "despairing anxiety" of the depressed phase in combination with the flight of ideas and feeling of internal pressure of the manic state. I have seen this rage emerge in children as young as 4.

---

### Ten Markers of Bipolar Disorder in a Child's Rage

*Rage is a predominant feature of early-onset BD and has 10 distinctive markers when seen in the behavior of elementary-school-age boys and girls.*

1. **The child may be fine at school during the day.**
   The rage happens at home, at night during rebound from medication when exhaustion from the effort of controlling herself all day overwhelms the child's ability to cope. The child is most vulnerable to rage late afternoon after school.[39]

2. **The rage may erupt for "no apparent reason."**
   Sometimes, it appears as if the child's rage comes out of nowhere, with parents and teachers at a loss as to what caused the outburst. At other times, the child's rage is in response to being denied something (e.g., told "no") or to some prohibition being put on his/her behavior. While being denied something or being told "no" are identifiable reasons, the child's reaction is extreme given the oftentimes-benign requests that are made by others. This "sudden explosive" quality is signatory of early-onset BD.

3. **Once activated, the rage takes a predictable course through build-up, explosive behavior, and diminution.**
   The child often reports headaches or exhaustion, or goes to sleep after the rage episode.

4. **The volume of the rage is great.**
   According to Dr. Charles Popper, bipolar-related rage is so powerful that "you could not imitate it if you tried."[40] The child may rave,

---

giggle, cry, and shout obscenities. He may lose all coping skills and emotionally regress to a much younger age.

5. **Gory thinking involving the use of knives, fire or dismemberment of loved ones is often verbally expressed by the child during rage.**
Rarely does the child follow through on threats, but the intensity of the delivery can be terrifying.

6. **The child attacks and destroys prized objects.**
He also goes after his parents' things, throwing the remote at the answering machine or chucking the pepper mill through the dining room.

7. **The child describes the rage as a buildup of heat, a seizure-like feeling.**
This involves the front side of the body, from the stomach, the sternum, the throat, the face, to the head. Some children report an aura before the buildup of rage, visual fuzziness, a waking "bad dream," sensitivity to smells, or headaches.

Anecdotal evidence from my clients and some research suggests that mania in BD may share many of the features of a brain seizure. In a seizure, loss of consciousness occurs, accompanied by involuntary motor muscle movements. This is caused by brain neurons firing randomly over an area of the brain that has been damaged by trauma, or a result of disease – a brain scar will "light up" when a seizure is viewed with brain scan technology.

The theory that manic-depression and seizures are related is strengthened by the fact that when children with early-onset BD experience rage, they may show several physical changes that also occur to a child who is in the midst of a brain seizure. These effects include a loss of awareness that may be severe enough to stop a child in his tracks, totally without a clue as to who he is or what he is doing. Becoming enraged, his pupils may dilate. Afterwards, he may have amnesia of what he did during the rage episode.

My clinical experience leads me to believe that kids who have these seizure-like effects are the most severe cases of early-onset BD. A caveat is in order: The presence of these symptoms is not diagnostic of the presence of BD but does indicate that at some level the brain is going through physical as well as psychological change when bipolar symptoms become florid.[41]

8.  **Children report rage almost as an entity that takes them over or that is clearly localized as a presence.**
    *"It's like the Donald Duck cartoon in which the devil (rage) sits on my left shoulder and the angel on the right."* One of my clients reported it as *"my brain (rage) vs. my heart (her family)."* This girl had intuitively localized the demon in her limbic brain and felt caught in a crossfire between it and the rest of her world.

9.  **Nothing satisfies the child's demands.**
    *Nothing is good enough. The child seems unable to derive a sense of reward from any activity. Even things like a prized stuffed animal that could give him pleasure when he is in a good mood, no longer comfort him. This increases his misery and he may attack them as if they have betrayed him, tearing them into pieces. He is unable to experience pleasure from anything (a phenomenon referred to as "anhedonia").*
    *This profound anhedonia is expressed in the destruction of comfort objects such as teddy bears. Some children challenged by BD experience a sense of relief from their chronic anhedonia by the release of adrenaline that causes release of pleasure neurochemicals in the brain, such as encephalin or enkephalin.*

10. **Rage may be treated effectively with anticonvulsant medication or the newer generation of anti-psychotics.**
    *Rage may be made worse by treatment with the antidepressant class of medications such as Prozac, Luvox, or Lexapro.*[42]

---

***Meltdown.*** Meltdown, a term popularized by Dr. Ross Greene in his book *The Explosive Child,* is a powerful emotional event, but is not as severe as rage. Meltdown is a temper tantrum that occurs in reaction to anxiety. While meltdowns can occur in response to other emotional states aside from anxiety, for the purpose of this discussion, I am focusing primarily on anxiety. It is typically pushed by the child's inability to cope with some outside stressor rather than by an eruption of emotional energy in his limbic system.

Children with AS experience frequent meltdowns brought on by the intense frustration they experience in getting their everyday needs met. They may have a difficult time understanding what is said to them (as is seen in a child who experiences auditory processing problems), or they may find it impossible to read and understand emotional nonverbal behavior. They may experience a right-brain learning disorder (see Chapter Three for a discussion of nonverbal learning disorder), and have difficulty doing math, understanding what they read, or solving abstract problems. Not being able to process information can be extremely distressing because the child feels cut off from help just when he needs it most. The result is a powerful and regressed loss of self-control – a meltdown.

---

### Eight Characteristics of Meltdown

1. ***It is an avoidant reaction.***
   *The child screams, holds his ears, and runs away. Or, if he attacks an adult, he pulls his punches. Unlike rage that is often very aggressive, meltdown is an attempt to escape from a stressor. A child with AS or autism may scream during a meltdown as a way to provide a kind of "white noise" soothing of his internal distress.*

2. ***The child may hurl invectives but there is a frantic quality to her swearing – it is sensed as angry frustration.***
   *The child will not report that temper dyscontrol felt activating as will a child diagnosed with BD.*

3. ***Meltdown is often triggered by an adult's attempt to gain compliance, such as to require the child to complete a lesson at school.***
   *Unlike rage related to BD, which may be triggered by the adult saying "No" to some demand the child makes, in my observation meltdown is triggered by adults trying to push the child to do something he does not want to do.*[43]

4. ***Meltdown may be triggered by interruption of an obsession.***
   *This cause can be hard to identify because, although the child may nonverbally express great frustration, he does not talk about its source. When a meltdown is related to the interruption of an obsession, the child may seem inner-focused, staring down to the front as his control disintegrates. He is trying to recover the obsession and complete it.*

   *Children with BD may experience rage when they are interrupted in the performance of an obsession or compulsion. This is why it is important to look closely at other diagnostic features and resist the temptation to say, "He throws such huge and disturbing temper fits.*

---

*I know he's bipolar!" It is an important question: Is he becoming intimidated and striking out to protect himself (meltdown) or is he "prosecuting the attack"? to use the military term for strategically attacking someone for advantage.*

*Confounding the difficulty in assessing for the presence of meltdown is the fact that children with AS also have meltdowns if they don't get their way. And they have meltdowns when getting their way is required to fulfill an obsession. It is important to look at all the other factors when trying to decide if you are dealing with the rage of a child afflicted with BD or the terror of a child with OCD and AS.*

5. **Meltdown may result from oversensitivity to some stimulus or a misperception of a social situation.**
   *The former could include a particular noise, an adult's tone of voice, or being in a crowded place with other children. The latter would involve the child incorrectly believing that a teacher is mocking him in front of other kids in the class.*

6. **A child may experience a meltdown when an adult tries to change his position on an issue.**
   *The child is very stubborn (e.g., "inflexible), totally fixed on her own way of looking at the situation and becomes extremely distressed when her perspective is countered by another person.*

7. **Meltdown may result from poorly planned transitions at school or home.**
   *Changing stimuli from being in a different setting is sensed as extremely disturbing to the child.*

8. **Because meltdown expresses the child's high anxiety, medication used to treat anxiety in the antidepressant class often reduces the explosivity of meltdown.**
   *Medications such as Luvox, Celexa, or Paxil may be used for this purpose.[46]*

## The Look and Feel of AS Plus BD

The following discussion will focus on 14 dimensions of the personality of children challenged by AS plus BD. I have put together this list of features from my own experience as a counselor with this population and from relevant research studies, which are cited.

### Features of the AS-plus-BD Neurotype

1. **Mood swing**

   Children with AS as a stand-alone diagnosis have a tendency to get depressed, and their mood may swing from normal to mild depression with stress. They are usually not impulsive at these times, but act anxious and withdrawn. Mania or hypomania are not part of the AS neurotype. If mania is present, the child will also meet the criteria for BD. Mania in these kids typically expresses itself very much like the mania seen in neurotypical elementary-age kids, but it will be less informed by common sense.

   Lack of common sense is evidenced by the fact that children with the AS-plus-BD presentation are less able to understand the impact of their behavior on themselves and others, and are less able to self-manage hypomania or mania. Children with BD alone understand the relationship between not taking medication and the onset of mania that may happen within hours of a missed dose of meds. They will be able to sense the onset of mania and call for help.

   Children with AS typically have a more difficult time "remembering" that they are manic and have less understanding of the impact of their behavior while manic. During a manic episode, one AS-plus-BD teen drank antifreeze to "see if he could survive." When asked if he knew that even if he did survive he might have been blinded for life, he answered, "I wasn't sure if that would happen or not." The disordered thought process demonstrated in this response (being blinded was an acceptable risk of the experiment) reflects the profound lack of common sense of the AS neurotype.[47]

   When a child is challenged by AS plus BD, his AS-related inability to figure things out is combined with his mood disorder, which magnifies the worst aspects of the mood disorder: He is less able to control his impulsivity, and rage. In teens, the depressed aspect may be expressed in hypersomniac retardation – the upset in sleep-wake rhythm described above. Children with the AS-plus-BD neurotype express mania with destructive impulsivity, staying up all night or compulsively hyperfocusing on a special interest.[48]

Dr. Lorna Wing followed a series of individuals with AS through puberty. Of these, 23% showed signs of affective illness, 11% had attempted suicide, and 17% were psychotic.[49]

## 2. Inheritability

A survey of my client families shows that both conditions have a similar pattern of heritability as stand-alone diagnoses. I have observed a slightly greater preponderance of families with AS-plus-BD children in which the mother carries traits of BD in her family line and the father carries traits of AS or HFA.

## 3. Psychosis

This is one of the most common and frightening features of the AS-plus-BD type. Psychosis is not a characteristic feature of AS. The psychotic states – hallucinations, extreme mania, and thought distortion – of BD are a major challenge for any child with BD as a stand-alone diagnosis, but the presence of common sense makes it possible to manage psychotic ideation. In the combined neurotype, however, the child tends to be more isolated in his delusions and more prone to suicidal ideation and destructive impulsivity. For example, he may get into dangerous experimentation with chemicals or electricity and inhabit the "mad scientist" archetype.

On the other hand, "mild" psychosis may contribute to the child's creative genius, giving him unbridled energy in the pursuit of his creative dreams. Observe the lives of great inventors, such as the very Asperger-like Nikola Tesla, inventor of AC/DC current. In Tesla's writings and life, you see great inventive genius but also personal "battiness," fascination with the weird and bizarre, and very poor self-care. These are characteristics of people who from time to time experience psychotic states.[50]

### 4. Rage, not meltdown

The child with the combined diagnosis experiences temper dyscontrol as rage, not meltdown. He is more aggressive than he would be if BD were not part of the picture. He is also less responsive to strategies used to avoid rage, such as self-report of feelings state, and he is isolated and miserable between episodes.

The DSM-IV considers "a distinct period of abnormally irritable mood" to be a manifestation of mania. I believe that the rage of an elementary-school-aged child with BD expresses mania this way. Later, in adolescence, this manic irritability may be expressed with chronic, verbally and physically abusive behavior. Tinged with the depression inherent in the condition, it may also be self-destructive, such as when a BD-challenged adolescent grabs the holstered weapon of a police officer and threatens to kill him.

### 5. Attention

Upwards of 90% of children with the diagnosis of BD have problems with inattention and distractibility. This marked inattention may be caused by their experience of flight of ideas. That is, their thought process is sped up so fast that they cannot pay attention to new stimuli. Inattention, distractibility, and memory problems are also characteristic of children with AS and HFA, but in these kids these issues are not related to pressured thought. More often, they express an impaired memory function, difficulty understanding emotion-based language, or a hyperfocus on irrelevant details (e.g., stimulus overselectivity). Complicating this attentional process may be hypervigilance – putting so much energy into anticipating attack that the child is not thinking clearly.

### 6. Social skills and interpersonal orientation

Children with BD may be clever, determined, and quite effective in getting what they want from others. Children with AS, on the other hand, do not typically show good language pragmatics or social pragmatics in general. This means that they do not understand the ordinary rules of conversation and are clumsy, one-sided, and rude in their attempts to communicate with others. Socially, they do not understand the rules for polite interaction; a 20-year-old college student, for example, may not understand that it is not O.K. to wear his underwear in the dorm room when his roommates have girlfriends visiting. I use the term "poor pragmatics" to denote this lack of common sense.

Research indicates that both children with BD and children with autism and AS have a difficult time decoding the emotional states and intentions of others. Specifically, children with BD tend to interpret facial expressions denoting happy, fearful, and sad as angry in all three cases.[51]

### 7. Common sense and self-care

Children and adolescents with BD can be very impractical in the hypomanic stage. Younger children are apt to hurt themselves with destructive impulsivity or in a rage. Teens get into trouble with excessive pleasure-seeking or make grandiose and unattainable plans, and they have splits that are more distinct between their elevated and depressed mood states.

If AS-plus-BD challenges the child, her common sense will be even more deficient. She will be drawn to danger but will be less capable of dealing with it than would be the case if her only issue were the presence of BD. Conversely, children with BD can be very clever in the pursuit of their goals.[52]

I have observed that children in the AS-plus-BD type are better able to take care of themselves in strange and novel situations. They take more risks and learn more from that impetus. The presence of hypomania makes them more aggressive and less passive when faced with threats from other children.

### 8. Learning disabilities

Executive function problems, very common in ADD and AS, include difficulty with self-organization, short-term memory, distractibility, and inattention. These factors are also seen in depressed children but they come in with the depression and fade when the depression lifts. They are chronic and lifelong conditions for many kids with ADD and AS.

In the AS-plus-BD presentation, the drop into depression, which crashes the cognitive process, may complicate these learning problems. For example, the child may become depressed in the middle of a test and, therefore, is unable to finish it. If the child is obsessing on some grievance (a typical challenge for children with BD), his attention will collapse and enhance the power of his AS to pull him into his own world around the issue. At this point learning ceases.

Assessment of learning disabilities in both AS and BD is complicated by the fact that both conditions tend to come with high IQ. The tester's office may be pleasantly challenging to both neurotypes for different reasons, and in this safe environment, the child's learning problems may not appear. She is totally tuned in and as resourceful as she can be.[53]

9. **Obsessive-compulsive thoughts**

In the AS-plus-BD neurotype, the tendency for both conditions to be obsessive and perfectionist come together to increase the force of the obsessive demand. It becomes much harder for the child to resist obeying the command. Younger children devolve into rage because their obsessions are interrupted or because caregivers do not comply with an obsessive demand. Teens may become delusional in the pursuit of an obsession – teens will not share the thought that is driving or bothering them. Evidence from my practice suggests that children and teens with the AS-plus-BD presentation are more susceptible to disorders that cross the line between OCD and psychosis, such as anorexia and the practice of self-cutting. They are intensely curious about extreme states of feeling and may hurt themselves in the pursuit of extreme experience.

10. **Sleep problems**

Children in the AS-plus-BD combination show abnormalities in circadian rhythm characteristic of BD. Though insomnia and nighttime cognitive hyperactivity are not characteristic of children and teens with AS, in combination with BD, they may show a tendency to be extreme night persons. My AS-plus-BD clients often tell me that they love to go out into the cool night air to enjoy the absence of people and the visually refreshing tones of black and white. Unfortunately, sleep deprivation causes both a hyper-energized state and a drop in cognitive ability. As a result, they may do very foolish things in these night ramblings and the next day may show hypersomniac retardation, the dull-mindedness seen in the demeanor of many children with the combined neurotype.

## 11. Sexuality

Children with BD may be hypersexual and may express these feelings impulsively. In the BD-plus-AS neurotype, the child's BD-derived sexual proclivities may be expressed from a very early age. Typically, the child's behavior does not evidence presence of sexual excitement with these acts as they would in adults but shows a kind of mindless impulsivity or compulsivity. The child just has to do the behavior, cannot stop herself, and does not know why.[54]

For example, an enraged 7-year-old will slap his mother's breasts and make vulgar sexual remarks to her. A middle-school-aged child may inappropriately touch a girl, not knowing that this behavior is considered offensive and dangerous – his AS-related problem with pragmatics retards his ability to understand why his actions are considered assaultive.

## 12. Substance use

One recent study documented substance abuse in 60% of adolescents with BD surveyed who were diagnosed with Bipolar I and in 50% of those diagnosed with Bipolar II hypomania, but not mania.[55] If they do become addicted, children with the AS-plus-BD presentation may show an inability to understand the consequences of substance use. As a result, they are not good candidates for substance abuse treatment programs such as that developed by Alcoholics Anonymous, which use a conceptual and abstract treatment model.

Many of my adolescent clients with the dual diagnosis smoke cigarettes. My guess is that this is partially self-medication. Nicotine raises dopamine levels dramatically in the short term and may be sought out to offset the painful inability to focus on things that goes with the AS-plus-BD neurotype. Smoking causes a momentary improvement in cognitive ability and makes an odd kid "one of the crowd." Unfortunately, cigarette smoking makes mood shift worse. Nicotine is a powerful drug, and the human brain is amazingly receptive to its use (there are actually nicotinic neurotransmitter receptors). The withdrawal and craving that happens many times a day as a result of smoking is a hugely destabilizing force in the child's personality.

## 13. Physical and emotional aggressiveness

Children with AS are less apt to display initiative in the expression of anger; that is, they are less apt to physically attack others and pursue the attack while in meltdown mode. Besides, they are not effective in delivering the attack. If they are not angry, they are characteristically passive.

A child with the AS-plus-BD neurotype is usually aggressively insulting when he is enraged and may use objects to attack his parents' property or persons. He may nurse a grievance against someone at school and plot ways to get even, or he may use the genius expressed in his special interest (computers, for example) to attack a source of his grievance (the school district's computer system). Children with AS-plus-BD who have poor control over their aggressive impulse may become threats to themselves and others and be very much at risk because they do not have the common sense to pull back and take a deep breath when this is the best thing to do.

## 14. Suicidality

Suicide is a huge risk factor for the child with the AS-plus-BD diagnosis. In their seminal work, *Manic Depressive Illness*, Goodwin and Jamison put the completed suicide rate for people with manic depression at 15 to 20%.[56] In another study, Dr. Barbara Geller and colleagues determined that better than 25% of children and adolescents diagnosed with BD had attempted suicide.[57]

The bipolar predilection for "solving" a personal problem this way is compounded by the AS tendency to withdraw into self under stress and lack of understanding of the countersuicidal messages provided by caregivers. Children with AS do not have practical ways of dealing with these powerfully painful thoughts. They cannot look at things with a little "common sense." These forces add up to increase the probability that a troubled AS-plus-BD teen will attempt to kill himself.

## Issues of Dual Diagnosis for Elementary-Age Children and Adolescents

| Feature | BD | AS/PDD | Combined Type |
|---|---|---|---|
| 1. Mood swing | From hypomania to depression; very impulsive in hypomanic phase | Chronic depression in which the child may be sad, irritable, oppositional, and verbally aggressive. Impulsivity not common | Extreme mood states and rapid cycling, obsessionality, and presence of special interest[58] |
| 2. Heritability of condition | Yes. A 40% chance if a first-degree relative is diagnosed with BD | Yes. A 40% chance if a parent is diagnosed with AS | Slightly better chance of expression if mother's line carries BD and father's AS |
| 3. Psychotic states | • Visual and auditory hallucinations<br>• Thought disorder | Not characteristic | • Dangerous isolation<br>• Severe thought disturbance; may be expressed in special interest |
| 4. Rage and meltdown | Rage, which occurs predominantly in younger children; less often in adolescents | Meltdown, not rage in younger children | Rage triggered by sensory overload and delusions |
| 5. Attention | • Severe distractibility caused by flight of ideas and hypomania<br>• Loss of function in depressed phase | • Chronic distractibility<br>• Inattention<br>• Memory problems | Cognitive problems made worse by emotional overwhelm |

## Issues of Dual Diagnosis for Elementary-Age Children and Adolescents

| Feature | BD | AS/PDD | Combined Type |
|---|---|---|---|
| 6. Social skills and interpersonal orientation | • Tendency to be dominant, controlling and aggressive, or have social phobia<br>• May anticipate harm from others<br>• In "flight" manifestation of BD, socially withdrawn | • Lack of a "theory of mind"<br>• Lack of repertoire of social skills<br>• Not typically aggressive<br>• Poor language pragmatics | • No, or few, friends<br>• School refusal<br>• Harmful anticipation<br>• Bullying others |
| 7. Common sense and self-care | Very goal-directed but self-defeating in hypomanic stage | Poor common sense, somewhat naive and passive | Takes dangerous risks uninformed by common sense |
| 8. Learning disabilities | • Not characteristic<br>• Performance sabotaged by emotional issues | • Central auditory processing problems<br>• Nonverbal learning problems (reading nonverbal behavior and solving problems) | LDs complicated by depression and difficulty learning compensatory strategies |
| 9. OCD | Frequent, express hypervigilance | Common, mild; difficult to separate from more general anxiety issues | • Severe<br>• Anorexia not uncommon |
| 10. Sleep problems | Virtually diagnostic in children who activate when it gets dark and stay awake all night | Not characteristic unless the child is obsessing | • Active insomnia<br>• Report that they enjoy absence of stimulation at night and opportunity for solitary undisturbed thought<br>• Report enjoyment of muted colors and cooler temperature at nighttime |

**Issues of Dual Diagnosis for
Elementary-Age Children and Adolescents (continued)**

| Feature | BD | AS/PDD | Combined Type |
|---|---|---|---|
| 11. Sexuality | Hypersexuality is not uncommon from an early age; inappropriate touching | Typically low level of interest in sex. In danger because of naiveté | • Under the age of 10, sexually dysinhibited<br>• Tendency for angry asexuality, hypermorality in adolescence |
| 12. Substance use | Common; 57% substance abuse rate | Rare. In danger because of naiveté when substance use is present; AA does not work | Cigarette addiction common – worsens mood shift |
| 13. Aggressiveness | Severe, almost definitive of condition in children and teens | Flight not fight; passive not aggressive | May attack property, be verbally threatening, show poor problem solving |
| 14. Suicidality | Severe risk | Not characteristic | Severe risk. May be severely depressed and lack ability to reframe depressing thoughts toward any positive outcome |

## Positive Aspects of the AS-plus-BD Neurotype

There are some archetypal patterns of strength in each diagnosis. I use the word "archetype" to describe common patterns of personality that I have observed in children with different diagnoses. Some readers may be familiar with the "Hunter" archetype, popularized by writer Thom Hartmann to describe the ever-inquisitive and energized ADD personality.[59]

I propose that children diagnosed with BD fit the "Warrior" archetype, to describe their aggressive and dominance-oriented natures (as well as their strengths in courage and capacity to use their skills to protect others). And I use the term "Scientist" or "Hermit" to describe the archetype of the child with AS as a potential wisdom-bringer to culture.

The child with BD is as courageous as she is willful. She is used to going to the extremes of physical and emotional endurance. The child with AS or HFA is intensely curious about how things function and how they interact in systems. She may be a natural at changing or streamlining the way something works because she is capable of intense, focused perspective. She may be an inventive genius.

Put these archetypes together and you see the potential. One example is embodied in the persona of luminaries like the great Bach interpreter Glenn Gould, who died in 1982. Gould showed aspects of HFA or AS in his single-minded devotion to the interpretation of Bach on the piano, his inability to relate to others, his obsessionality, and his sensory integration issues. His behavior also showed evidence of the experience of hypomania – he did not sleep for days but roamed the streets of Toronto in his black Cadillac going nowhere in particular. He experienced powerful depressive states as well as states of unbridled joy, such as when he took to running through the Toronto Zoo singing to all the animals.

Thomas Edison is another candidate for the AS-plus-BD label – an inventive genius with a mean streak. Edison would sleep an hour a night, on the average; he rarely changed his clothes, he was a slave driver as a manager, and his people skills were horrible. In addition, he had over 1,700 patents in his name. It is conceivable that his AS-related fascination for the perfect pattern in electrical design was complemented by the will and drive of a bipolar condition. Adults challenged by AS-plus-BD are very self-centered and have an air of "absent-minded professor" on hyperdrive.

Dr. Ted Kazcynski, the "Unabomber," may be a candidate for the dark side of the AS-plus-BD neurotype. Kazcynski, a mathematical genius and rising star at the University of California, showed many features of autistic-spectrum people. He had a metronomic habit of rocking, had extremely poor social skills and no friends, frequent concerns about germs, extremely poor personal hygiene, and seemed incapable of sympathy for other human beings. He was known as a "walking brain" at the university where he worked. Poor personal hygiene, obsessionality, and lack of empathy are features frequently seen in BD, but the most telling indications of the presence of mania in Kaczynski's personality were his "manifestos," the rambling, nonstop rants he would demand be published in various newspapers.[60]

## Five Strategies for Helping the AS-Plus-BD Child at Home

Much of this chapter has been devoted to describing the challenges of children with the combined diagnosis, but as we have just seen, there are also
powerful positives in the character of these children – positive aspects of
genius. No child ever got better because of hearing just the negative about
himself. The unique strengths in a child's personality must be recognized
and resourced if he is to achieve stability and success in life. Here are five
important strategies for helping these children realize their potential:

1. **Use mood charting to help you and your child identify and manage
   things that trigger his BD.**
   A mood chart is a record of the child's behavior on a day-to-day basis
   that helps you establish the presence of BD and manage the factors
   that bring it on. It does not have to be complicated or clinical to help
   you see patterns of BD in a child's behavior, mental activity, and emotional life.[61]

   You can make your own chart or browse online for a variety of different types. One useful format is found on the website for the Georgia
   Child Bipolar Foundation. You will need to download the Adobe Reader utility to acquire GCBF's chart (http://www.gcbf.org/hmm.pdf).

## Elements of a Typical Mood Chart[61]

| | |
|---|---|
| **Evidence of Mania** | Document the presence of unexpected changes in mood. Bipolar disorder affects children and teenagers differently, but there are features common to both age groups. Note behaviors that indicate the presence of distractibility, grandiosity, flight of ideas, pressured speech, hypersexuality, impulsivity, insomnia, and other indicators of mania. Consult the guidelines above for a description of mania in children and teens. |
| **Evidence of Depression** | Document the presence of these common features: (a) drop in the ability to do homework or ability to get up in the morning or go to school; (b) complaints of unbearable fatigue and lethargy; (c) suicidal statements or gestures; (d) depressed mood, sadness, and low self-esteem; and (e) changes in sleep or eating patterns; sleeping during the day and staying up all night, eating much more or much less than usual. Also, look for loss of interest in previously enjoyed activity, especially his "special interest."<br><br>Also, note these features of depression specific to age group. For teens, (a) self-destructive behavior such as picking fights with kids at school who will beat them up; (b) evidence of substance use; and (c) evidence of risky sexual behavior. Younger children are more apt to express the depressive stage with angry withdrawal, school refusal, and separation anxiety – they cannot tolerate being away from their mothers. |
| **Rage History** | Mark the days that rage occurred and length of each rage event. Note any obvious causative factors ("He was told we would not buy him the video game he wanted") and the most severe damage that resulted from the rage ("He hit his mother"). |
| **Causative Factors for Emergence of Symptoms** | Note probable causative factors; that is, trigger events that seem to push a drop in mood (see discussion of the "trigger situation list" below for more detail). Document any changes in routine, or failures at school or in social relationships that may bring on a mood shift. Look closely at the child's sleep patterns; mood instability follows sleep deprivation. Family conflict may also cause the onset of bipolar cycling. Note these stressors, to include arguments in the family – between parents or siblings – that are "heating" the emotions in the family. |
| **Medication** | Keep a daily record of the medications the child was given, the dosage, and any side effects. A range of powerful medications are prescribed for children with BD, including the antipsychotic class of drugs. Before switching medications, build a good medication history for your doctor's analysis of the effectiveness of a particular drug. Compare and contrast your analysis of your child's daily medication with the causative factors you noted under Rage History. It is important to understand if some outside stressor is overwhelming the ability of the medication to work or if it is the wrong med, or the correct med in the wrong dosage. Make sure to take into account the impact of stress in your child's life before judging the effectiveness of a particular medication. Stress brings out the worst in people, and it will exacerbate your child's symptoms. |

2.  **Use the "mood shift warning list" and "trigger situation list" to help your child manage mood shifts.**

    Children challenged by BD can benefit from the use of two personal inventories that keep a record of their emotional swings and point to ways to improve the situation: a mood shift warning list and a trigger situation warning list.

### *Mood Shift Warning*

The mood shift warning list is developed by the child to help her identify what physical and emotional signs preceded mood shift, such as loss of appetite, having compulsive thoughts, or a cessation of physical self-care. This strategy, described in my book *Survival Strategies for Parenting Children with Bipolar Disorder*, is one of the tools I use in my psychotherapy practice.[62]

---

**A Typical AS-Plus-BD Mood Shift Warning List**
**for Depression (for a Teenage Boy):**

*When my mood is shifting,*
I wake up feeling tired and crabby.

*As my mood darkens,*
I get more obsessive than usual.

*When I'm really into it,*
I can't get out of bed and sleep all day.

**For mania or hypomania ...**

*When my mood is shifting,*
I start listening to my crazy friends' advice to do stupid things.

*As my mood begins to become hypomanic,*
I stay up all night on the computer.

*When I'm really into it,*
I feel pleasantly angry all the time.
I am apt to do dangerously impulsive things.

---

### The Trigger Situation Warning List

The trigger situation warning list categorizes the stressors that may bring on a mood shift, such as staying up all night or breaking up with a girlfriend. These lists were written keeping in mind the unique challenges of children with AS-plus-BD.

---

**Trigger Situation Warning List**
*(These activities push mood shift)*

- Staying up all night
- Sneaking out with Mickey at school for a cigarette or puff of pot
- Disappointment
- Getting up too fast in the morning
- Drinking coffee at night and staying up late
- Eating sugar or not eating enough good food
- Any kind of big change
- Letting homework pile up – too much homework
- Being verbally abused by the kids at school
- Staying in the sun too long or riding my bike without a break
- My parents putting me down
- My parents fighting

Adapted from Lynn, G.T. (2000). *Survival strategies for parenting children with bipolar disorders*, p. 89. London: Jessica Kingsley Publishers. Reprinted with permission.

---

You may have to be very directive in helping your AS-plus-BD child keep and use these lists. I have learned from my work with these kids that they are not easily self-reflective and they are generally disorganized. It takes quite a bit of practice for them to learn to use tools such as these. Kids with HFA and AS have difficulty future pacing their behavior and do not intuitively understand cause and effect.

3. **Understand the importance of family connection and stability for symptom remission.**

   Practice good communication. Research with families who have members with BD and schizophrenia indicates that family instability and family communication patterns have a lot to do with whether a child experiences symptoms of BD. For example, this research indicates that a child's mood will destabilize into depression if his family is continually embroiled in struggle and argument, and his mood will destabilize into *mania* following the use of drugs or sleep deprivation. Other studies indicate that instability of any kind may prompt the on-set of symptoms in manic-depressive illness.[63] At the same time, this research makes it clear that there are things we can do to help a child avoid symptoms and things that we do that make things worse. Brain chemistry and environment are both implicated in lessening or worsen-ing symptoms.

We make things better by improving the way we communicate with each other and the child. Positive nonverbal behavior such as smiling at the child approvingly, giving her time to say her piece, and verbal encourage-ment go a long way in helping a child prone to mood shift stay in a good mood. Conversely, name-calling and yelling have a negative influence. This is not to say that the AS-plus-BD child does not contribute to the unpleasant uproar herself. She does. However, given the unfairness of this fact, it is up to caregivers to change things for the better. Here are three essential features of this kind of positive communication.

- *Listen with awareness of the child's impairment.* Do not take on ev-ery challenge and insult the child throws at you. Do not take it per-sonally and insist that the child behave with civility because "that is our family value." Good listening means that you do not lecture but try to find out what the child is experiencing. Work with him to identify what he wants and then help him get it in such a way that others are not hurt. Speak from an "I" position, simply identifying your feelings and beliefs without blaming or beating him up with his diagnosis – "You're the messed-up one here because you are bipolar! Did you remember to take your medication?"

- *Do not tolerate law breaking and abuse.* Let these acts have their natu-ral consequences. Though children with AS-plus-BD are less apt to get into trouble with the law (they lack the aggressiveness of the child with BD as a stand-alone issue), they may get violent at home and may physically attack family members. This is a time to call 911. It is also a time to call 911 when any evidence of law breaking is discovered. Pain-ful as it is, it is best to get the authorities involved sooner than later. In most cases, the nasty experience of arrest and possible requirement for community service will be the child's consequence.

- *If verbal abuse is a problem, practice a low-trust attitude toward privileges.* Let the child know the language that you consider to be "over the line." Then tell him that you will impose take-backs on any privileges he regularly enjoys if he insults you. Let him know that the family is a community; you put things in and you take things out. In his case, he has taken something out (your peace of mind and dignity) and, therefore, needs to give back or lose something as a result. Make a list of all the things that he derives from being a part of the family and consider making anything on the list, short of his health and safety, conditional. Stick to your guns. The AS-plus-BD character type looks for results. If your child does not find you true to your word, he will push harder to get his way. Also notice the positive in his demonstration of greater respect for you and reward it. This sends a signal that he is worthy of having greater leeway. You might choose to let him play his video game in bed at night until lights out. Or, for a teen, get an O.K. to go to a paint-ball meet. Greater parental trust in a child's choice of music, video games, and personal attire signal that he is an accepted member of the family community.

4. **Practice proactive and effective management of *rage* events at home.** Our discussion of the rage of children with AS-plus-BD does not capture the intensity of the experience for a child and his caregivers. An enraged child is truly "mad" in the classic sense of the word.

   My clinical experience is that rage becomes much less of a problem once a child with the dual diagnosis grows into puberty. As a teen, she may have very scary temper tantrums, but she has more control over these states. As a caveat, I would say that the children I see in my private practice are not drawn from an institutionalized population that would include more profoundly affected children. Still, anecdotal accounts and some survey research suggest that destructive pleasure-seeking and impulsivity is a greater problem than episodic rage for adolescents challenged by BD.[64]

   Getting the correct medication is the first order of business in rage management. Rage is a neurological event akin to a seizure. And, the enraged child is dangerous, impulsive, and potentially psychotic. We noted in our discussion of rage in BD that drugs in the anticonvulsant class are the first line of treatment for BD. This class includes drugs suck as Depakote, Lithium, and Trileptal.

Many children experience relief from the pressure to rage from treatment with the new-generation neuroleptics such as Risperdal and Abilify. The neuroleptics are able to reduce the expression of rage as well as treat the psychosis that often is seen in BD. Although every child reacts differently to medication, the neuroleptics may also reduce extreme expression of the aggravating features of AS seen in the AS-plus child's obsessive fixation, depressive irritable manner and distorted thinking.

Typically, children eventually respond to the right medication but the experimentation needed to find the right balance of meds can be exhausting. Nevertheless, I encourage parents to keep looking and not give up seeking the correct pharmacology for their child.

> *Side effects are a major concern when using neuroleptic medication. These medications are associated with liver damage, kidney damage, diabetes mellitus, weight gain, and cognitive dulling.*
>
> *A standard caveat is that parents and teachers pay attention to the child and listen when he complains about medication side effects. It is easy to ignore the psychic pain that they may cause a child. This pain will come in the form of intense irritability or restlessness that cannot be expressed. The child will feel as if his motor is running with the brakes on all day and will not be able to sleep at night (or will miss the experience of the pleasant hypnogogic drop off into sleep).*

The distinction between rage and meltdown must be made carefully in choosing the appropriate medication. Rage, if present, is best treated with a mood stabilizer or neuroleptic. Meltdown, as an anxiety reaction, is best treated with drugs that soothe high anxiety and depression, such as the selective serotonin reuptake inhibitors (SSRIs).

The next table summarizes essential features of a rage management plan that you can use to guide the process of managing your child's rage events. It is important to have a plan because a child's rage may come out of nowhere, and without a plan you will be doing nothing but controlling the child's wild and aggressive behavior. A plan enables you to do the right thing at the right time. I revisit several of the points noted in this table later on in my discussion of strategies for managing the rage event itself.

---

### Home-Based Management Plan

*A good rage plan helps parents behave effectively during the rage event.*

- Parents agree on who will be in charge and agree to support each other, as do other emergency responders; whoever is dealing with the immediate situation is in charge.

- The child is enrolled with a counseling center and with a medical professional who can coordinate involuntary commitment to a psychiatric facility if needed.

- Parents have located the nearest hospital emergency room should a crisis psychiatric evaluation be required prior to commitment. If a child needs emergency psychiatric evaluation, 911 responders should know where the parents want them to take their child.

- A list of crisis contacts is maintained that includes phone numbers to call to get assistance, such as the child's therapist, psychiatrist, or crisis response staff.

- Parents agree on the point at which they will call 911, and the child is made aware that this option will be used if she becomes violent.

---

This section summarizes suggestions contained in *Survival Strategies for Parenting Children with Bipolar Disorder*[65] for managing a child's expression of rage at home. In general, these rage management strategies also apply at school.

Children with BD move through a sequence of four phases in the escalating expression of rage: dysphoric affect, provocation, explosion, and exhaustion. To effectively manage the situation, parents must be able to reduce stress and redirect the child at each step to reverse the process.

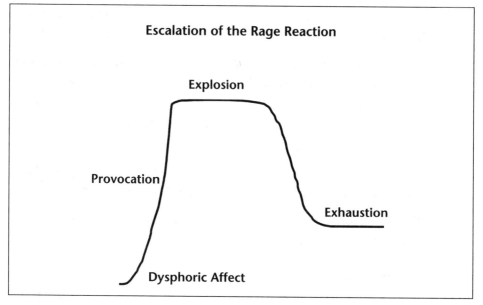

From Lynn, G. T. (2000). *Survival strategies for parenting children with bipolar disorder*, p. 60. London: Jessica Kingsley Publishers. Reprinted with permission.

## Dysphoric Phase

Rage often begins with the child's expression of bitter irritation. Everything annoys him and nothing comforts him. Behaviors characteristic of this phase include:

- Angry nonverbal facial expressions
- Raised voice
- Hyperactivity
- Pestering and whining
- Tormenting his parents with rude remarks, poking at his sister, bothering the cat

### Strategies for reducing dysphoria

- *Develop a check-in system with the child* such as the use of a color scheme to describe the buildup of angry tension – from "blue" (good mood) to "red" (angry, depressed mood). Another option is the 5-Point Scale developed by Kari D. Buron and Mitzi Curtis.[66]

- *Separate the child from stressful social situations.* If you see that she is warming up to a hassle with a friend, gently intervene and suggest separate activities. If possible, negotiate a resolution to the issue without being too obtrusive. Send the friend home if necessary.

- *Distract toward a calming pastime.* Suggest she go for a bike ride or ask her to run an errand for you with a reward for doing so. This is a good time to suggest exercise, which typically raises mood.

- *Offer her something to eat.* Blood sugar problems can worsen a child's mood and aggressive behavior.

## Provocative Phase

As the dysphoria deepens, the child begins to look around for a fight. The following behaviors are seen as he enters the provocative phase:

- A silly devilish facial expression

- Swearing and insults directed at other family members

- Interruption of parents' phone calls

- Threatening parents with making a scene

- Clenching fists and approaching parents using threatening nonverbal behavior

- Slamming doors

### Strategies for reversing provocative behavior

- *Call the game.* If the child seems to be following you around looking for a fight, say, "I have the feeling that you are trying to get a rise out of me for the fun of it. But I don't want to play that game. What can we come up with that would be more interesting for both of us?" Take the child's provocative behavior as her way of telling you that she is approaching her wit's end and needs some inspiration to keep from crashing into dysphoria and rage.

- *Avoid reacting.* Do not let the child goad you to angry reaction. Remember that at this point, her thinking capacity is reduced but her reactivity and sensitivity to your manner is greatly enhanced. She will see insult where there is none or feel provoked when you have done nothing to provoke her. This is the emergence of her fight-or-flight brain state and she may not be thinking clearly. Take a deep breath and remind yourself to stay calm. Keep breathing deeply, and you will stay in control.

- *Use positive, specific, and concise language* to help move the child away from provocative behavior. The general rule is that the child will do everything that comes after the word "Stop." Therefore, your statement to your child of "Stop teasing the dog" will result in an increase in the teasing behavior. Use positive language syntax. Do not say, "Pay attention!" Instead say, "I'll start again when you let me know that you want to talk and listen."

- *Use "reminder" language.* This can help because a child can lose awareness of her behavior in the heat of her provocation. For example, say, "When you show me that you are with me by no longer swearing at me but are talking politely, we can continue."

### Explosive Phase

At this point, the frontal lobes of the brain become functionally inoperative and the limbic brain takes over the child's behavior, catapulting him into total dysinhibition. The following behaviors occur:

- Screaming and crying, sometimes at the same time, sometimes with sufficient force to break facial blood vessels

- Foaming at the mouth, dilation of the pupils

- Clinically paranoid ideation. The child darts around the house furtively trying to avoid adults or accusing them of trying to do him harm

- Death threats against parents and siblings, suicide threats

- Threatening with knives, electrical appliances, and heavy objects

- Behaving violently toward pets – usually short of doing serious harm

- Wild evasive behavior, running into the street, attempting to jump out of a moving car
- Hitting and scratching parents

### Strategies for controlling the force of the explosive phase

This is the acute stage of the reaction. At this stage, the child is functionally unable to listen or follow corrective action. The appropriate strategy is to maintain firm boundaries while avoiding direct encounter with the child so that the explosive phase has time to run its course.

- *Do not argue with the child and do not overreact.* Do not give in. Enforce the rules that are important while trying to give the child some control of the outcome.
- *Use short words and short sentences.* Complex verbal messages will not be understood at this time. "Telegraph" your directives to the child and don't argue:
  - "Please go to your room now."
  - "Sit down and breathe slowly a couple of times."
  - "You are swearing at me. I will talk to you when the swearing stops."
- *Attend to your own stress.* Take a breath down to your diaphragm and remind yourself that you must be in control. Give yourself a few minutes away from the situation if you start losing your temper.
- *Protect other family members.* It is up to you to make sure that other children are physically safe and do not have to listen to the verbal abuse of the raging child. Implement arrangements you have made beforehand. Have them go to their rooms, lock their doors, and put on headphones and listen to favorite music.
- *Use restraint very selectively and very carefully.* Some parents choose to use physical restraint to control their child's dangerous behavior during the explosive phase. Restraint should only be used on young children (top of head no higher than a parent's chest). It should be used only to prevent the child from harming himself or somebody else. The only safe restraint hold is the "basket hold," a position in which the adult stands behind the child holding his hands and arms straight up without jerking on his arms. If a child

is too big for the basket hold, he is too big to be restrained in the home and parents should seriously consider calling emergency responders for help.

- *Call for back-up if needed.* Agree beforehand whether you will call 911 if violence occurs. Consider contracting with a local psychiatric facility that is set up to intake the child if he is brought to the hospital by police. Know that allowing the child to be violent with you breeds more violence. Do what you need to do to maintain strong boundaries on his rage dyscontrol.

## Exhaustion Phase

Children with rage related to early-onset BD demonstrate several characteristic behaviors when rage subsides:

- The child often collapses and appears dazed and "out of it"

- He complains of a bad headache

- He falls asleep for a period of time

- He does not remember what happened during the rage

- Upon waking, many children express genuine remorse for their actions or may refuse to talk about what happened. The child's denial is fueled by his terror that he is broken, crazy, incurable, and shameful

### Strategies for Using the exhaustion phase as an opportunity for healing

To help the child learn from her experience, do not counter or blame, but take a reflective stance. Simply mirror back any statements she might make about her feelings around the event. Briefly relate events from your own life that may be comparable to her experience. Let her talk. It is more important that she talk to you than it is for her to listen to your suggestions for change. If conversation proceeds naturally, you may get the opportunity to introduce and process the event. Use these questions to frame that discussion:

- What behavior did you believe was problematic?

- What is your concern or need?

- What set things off?

- What could we all do if this situation comes up again?

This is an opportunity for reflection, bridge building, and corrective action planning. It should result in affirmation of the child's intention to have more control in the future and build a feeling of "live and learn," of planning for a better future. The objective of this analysis is to create a positive climate for problem solving at home. This feeling of positive cooperation is important to helping the child maintain his mental stability. The message from parents must be: "We love you but do not and will not accept your destructive behavior."

There is a good chance that rage will occur again, and when it does, the child will not remember these good intentions. Do not expect his good intentions to change the situation but understand that cultivating the feeling of positive regard and acceptance does work toward reducing the frequency of reoccurrence of the event.

5. **Work with the child to co-create a positive Great Story.**
Given the present-moment orientation of kids with AS and HFA, it is difficult for a child to create and remember the vital personal narrative that answers so many important questions in her life, including the three big ones: "Who am I?" "Who are all these others?" and "What are we doing together?" Researchers such as Dr. Daniel Siegel have suggested that having a personal autobiography is also essential for neurological development.[67] To help the child form a positive story for her own life, make time every day to listen to her and weave in archetypal themes that are seen in the lives of people with the AS-plus-BD neurotype. Consider the "great persons in history theme." Tell the child that though her path in life may be difficult, there is good reason to believe that she was born with the personality features of people who moved the world with their accomplishments and discoveries. Help her see that sometimes "perfect happiness living the suburban life" is not for everyone and that being discontented is O.K.! Let her know that it is a myth that people can get through life unscathed by trouble and that she has the advantage of having trouble up-front when she is a kid, so that she will be better equipped to deal with

it later in life. Tell her that the "great bipolar geniuses of history" lived to follow their passions even though following their "bliss" in this way may have had a cost for them in terms of security and contentment.

The child challenged by AS-plus-BD lives in terror of not being able to control his mind. Assure him that by paying attention to his mood change and the impact of stress in his life, he can learn to anticipate and direct his mood shifts. Let him know that with proper lifestyle habits and the right medication, he has every chance of doing very well in life.

## Five Strategies for Helping the AS-Plus-BD Child at School

Though there are no statistics that predict high school completion rates for children with BD, there is a staggering 50% high school dropout rate for children classified as "emotionally disturbed," and BD is the diagnosis of some of those with the most serious impairments.[68]

This dismal completion rate is often a function of the poor fit between the standard structure of education and the bipolar neurotype. Although challenged by mood shift, a child with BD as a stand-alone condition may have intact, neurotypical thought processes. The child with the combined diagnosis must deal with both the limitations of mood dyscontrol stemming from BD and the learning problems, lack of common sense, and self-organization issues associated with AS. Creative approaches are needed to help kids with the more complex challenges of the AS-plus-BD type get an education so they live successful, satisfying, and self-sustaining adult lives.

The AS-plus-BD neurotype challenges children differently at different stages in the developmental process. Some elementary-school-age children are capable of holding down their bipolar-spectrum symptoms at school, but explode at the least provocation at home. They may not have learning problems but may, in fact, excel at school. Other children in this age group show consistent patterns of inattention that may be mistaken for ADD or AD/HD. These children are not helped by stimulant medication and may become agitated or withdrawn after taking it. They may be explosive at school and unreceptive to redirection.

Teens tend to drop into depressive funks, sleeping through their first period at school. They are drawn to highly stimulating activities and are prone to dangerous impulsivity with regard to drugs and sexual behavior, which will tend to be anonymous, experimental, and spontaneous. When their depressions hit, cognitive function ceases. They may be hyper-vigilant and very argumentative. More than half will be diagnosed with conduct disorder.[69] Some will gradually isolate themselves from others, becoming more reclusive and depressed. Many are addicted to nicotine. Withdrawal from nicotine, avoiding sleep at night, and drug withdrawal may all cause symptoms of mania or depression to emerge.[70]

1.  **Recognize the AS-plus-BD child at school.**
    (Excerpted in part from the website of the Child and Adult Bipolar Foundation. http://www.bpkids.org.)[71]

*Grades K Through 6*

- Is a loner on the playground; has no friends.

- May become hypomanic and giddy when required to perform tasks. This state may devolve into rage.

- Is highly anxious and refuses to go to school.

- Shows sensory integration problems (crowding, fluorescent lights, smells, and building noise are experienced as pain).

- Is given to destructive impulsivity, hitting other children, or running away from school.

- Is vocally hyperactive; does not listen.

- Voices negative self-esteem/muses about own death.

- May possess learning disabilities characteristic of the AS population, to include auditory processing problems, difficult forming abstractions, and high social anxiety.

- May possess gifts typical of both diagnoses such as the ability to apply intelligence to a special interest, powerful vocabulary, and IQ measured in the "very superior" range.

### Grades 7 Through 12

- Great difficulty getting up for first-period classes.

- May show severe social phobias.

- May be given to tearfulness and hyperemotionality.

- May show evidence of substance use.

- May be aggressive and hyper-reactive. In depressive phase may pick fights he cannot win.

- Isolated, quits activities, and does not show initiative.

- Becomes hypomanic and stays up all night, sleeps during day.

- Inflated self-esteem (will announce very unrealistic academic ambitions).

### Issues Common to the Child K-12 with the AS-Plus-BD Presentation[71]

- May report visual and auditory hallucinations.

- Sometimes experiences increased thirst, frequent urination, drowsiness, sluggishness, and other side effects of medication.

- Demonstrates severe fluctuations in energy and motivation.

- Becomes overheated and dehydrated from physical exertion on hot days.

- Acutely embarrassed when participating in team sports.

- Acutely embarrassed when speaking in front of others.

- Voices negative self-esteem/muses about own death.

2. **Provide a staff or volunteer in the role of "guiding hand" who understands children with the AS-plus-BD neurotype.**

   This recommendation holds for every neurotype in this book. The child with the AS-plus-BD presentation will need a person with a unique set of skills to help her get through the school day. These include the ability to stay calm and non-confrontive in the face of the child's rage and to help her develop more self-control. The "guiding hand" (GH) may or may not coordinate the child's IEP and behavior plan but should be a part of the IEP team. And, the person in this role should have the ability to also help the child in academic and social areas.

The unfortunate truth is that often the educational system does not follow through on the plans made at the IEP meeting. Given the bureaucratic nature of the system, it is unlikely that anything will happen unless someone on staff takes personal responsibility for the results. The GH makes sure things do not slip through the cracks. It is important that the GH be given the time and resources to do the job well.

3. **Implement the following 14 essential characteristics of an AS-plus-BD friendly educational setting.**

The IEP meeting is an opportunity to discuss the child's learning disabilities and behavior issues as well as his strengths. The team will have to wrestle with the predicament posed by the child's behavior. As a child with special needs, he should receive educational services, even if provided at private schools, that help him learn despite his impairment. However, if his behavior is hostile, bullying, or disruptive to other students, there may be pressure to put him in a restrictive classroom that serves children labeled "severe behavior disordered" or "emotionally disabled." Even though he may not be taught to his IQ level in the more restrictive environment, this may be seen as the only option given his emotional problems. In this case, his diagnosis trumps his IQ.

Depression in children with BD is made worse by stress caused by boredom and the humiliation of being labeled as psychiatric patients at school. This is why it is so important when looking at appropriate educational services for the AS-plus-BD child to make sure that the environment is not provoking her symptoms or that the teaching style is not making things worse. Some children with the dual diagnosis get along just fine at school if staff know how to avoid power struggles. Some children whose primary expression of BD is depression will be no problem at all in an active sense but will need help getting to school. Other children with the dual diagnosis will be provocative and problematic regardless of the academic setting they are in. Unfortunately, this latter group may track toward the self-contained, highly restrictive type of classroom.

It is important to understand that under the law the child's social and emotional development is as important as her academic progress. The school district cannot get out of providing services by saying "She's so smart. Look at her grades. She doesn't need an IEP." The district must take into account that the child's social and emotional difficulties may be challenging her stability at home and school and that these need to be addressed as well.

Here are some common features of the best learning environments for children with AS plus BD.

---

### To Teach the AS Plus BD Child

1.  *Provide teachers and staff with training on how to teach students with BD and AS.*

2.  *Place the student with AS-plus-BD with other emotionally vulnerable and fragile students, not with students whose behavior is the result of criminal or gang activities.*

3.  *Group the student with other intelligent, creative students when possible.*

4.  *Include the student's special interest in the curriculum and program science and art educational services around it.*

5.  *Make social skill development an integral part of the core curriculum.*

6.  *Plan a classroom routine that is predictable and structured.*

7.  *Monitor mood shifts and understand their impact on academics. Allow the student more slack when her cognitive capability is impaired due to mood instability, mania, or depression.*

8.  *In assessment, look for presence of nonverbal learning problems typical of the AS population. High verbal IQ may obscure the presence of other learning problems.*

9.  *Give the child a late-start schedule if needed to deal with morning somnolence. Schedule new or more challenging, cognitive material at mid-morning or early afternoon.*

10. *Be knowledgeable about medication side effects, such as increased thirst, frequent urination, drowsiness, and becoming easily overheated from exertion. For example, do not restrict the opportunity to use the drinking fountain or bathroom and do not require the child to take physical education classes.*

---

11. Provide staff with the name of an emergency contact person in addition to the parent to call if the student is vomiting, complains of severe abdominal pain or appears to be dehydrated. These are serious medication side-effect symptoms that need to be medically assessed.

12. Take dietary factors into account in scheduling classes. Allow time for lunch and snacks. Mood shift can be kicked off by blood sugar imbalance.[72]

13. Put in place an aggressive anti-bullying strategy and enforce it consistently.

14. Do not blame parents, but strive to work with them to help the child in his present placement or plan an alternative placement involving private contractors.

Use the following strategies to overcome learning disabilities typical of the AS-plus-BD child.

- Look for problems remembering and processing information provided verbally. If the student has a central auditory processing problem (i.e., difficulty understanding and acting on information communicated verbally), it is important to give him a visual record of all lessons.

- To deal with difficulty concentrating and remembering assignments, record the student's assignments daily in a notebook that is shared with parents. Have the GH monitor and keep this notebook up-to-date.

- Keep an eye out for dyslexia, a common learning disability among children challenged by BD. Implement teaching strategies and services from speech and language specialists to help the child learn.

**4. Practice proactive rage management at school.**

Designate staff who know their roles in the process and are trained in the procedure that will be used to manage rage events. They assist the classroom teacher in implementing the behavior management plan to maintain safety and de-escalate from crisis situations. It is important that all staff that are exposed to the child on a daily basis are aware of her issues and the impact of medication on the child's behavior and performance. They must accept the fact that the child is psychiatrically impaired and not blame her. They should get inservice training in de-escalation of rage that includes understanding when the child is "warming up" to temper dyscontrol and what to say and not say at this point. The list below summarizes key aspects of a rage management plan for a child with the dual diagnosis at school.

---

### Essentials of a School-Based Rage Management Plan

A behavior management plan should be in place that identifies:
1. Specific strategies the classroom teacher can use to cool down the situation.
2. What the teacher will do if the situation is not controlled (move all students to another classroom, escort child to principal's office or security, etc.).
3. Who will be called once the plan is initiated (IEP coordinator, school psychologist).
4. Who will take over the situation after the child leaves the classroom (principal, the school psychologist, or IEP coordinator).
5. At what point parents are called to come and get the child.
6. At what point 911 or campus security becomes involved.

---

Show teachers and other caregivers how to recognize the build-up toward rage. Use inservice training and conferences provided by parents and the child's mental health team to identify behavioral aspects of the warm-up to rage. Every child is different in this regard, but here are some potential markers:

- He has isolated himself from the other kids and seems to be looking around furtively or accusingly at others.

- He is glowering and showing signs of frustration with some project he is working on.

- He is becoming agitated, talking too fast, and his talk is becoming aggressive. He is beginning to move around the classroom knocking things off the other kids' desks.

All teaching, counseling, and administrative staff should know whom to call if the child's symptoms emerge. It is especially important to provide information to substitute teachers and bus drivers. In order to disseminate this information to all relevant staff, have the parents and child (if required by your state or province disclosure law) complete a release of information.

Know that the child needs strong boundaries *maintained by people who like him*. Remember that children with the AS-plus-BD neurotype who are in the provocative stage of the event are very sensitive to negative, angry, or rejecting feeling from adults in charge.

Use short words and short sentences that describe behavior. For example, say, "I will be glad to let you go back to class as soon as you show me you have control of your body."

Third, act (as one of my client parents put it) "like they do in psychiatric hospitals." Do not blow your cool. If you get upset, the child will cue to your feeling and enact this himself. Take a breath down to your diaphragm and remind yourself that you will eventually have control of the situation. Say to yourself, "Breathe now. Down to belly. Good. I am in charge. I will get through this. Breathe."

Write a detailed and clear behavior management plan that reduces the probability of rage at school by creating a school environment loaded for success. A psychologist or other expert trained to make such an assessment can do a functional behavior assessment (FBA) for the student. In the FBA, specifically identify the stressors that may push the child toward temper dyscontrol and the action staff can take to improve the situation. Then write a behavior management plan based on this assessment. The following table identifies some of the key aspects of a good plan.

## Key Aspects of a Behavior Management Plan for a 9-Year-Old Child with AS Plus BD with Features of Rage Dyscontrol

| | |
|---|---|
| 1. Identify his character strengths | • Loves anime; has written a computer program for drawing anime figures.<br>• Has demonstrated his personal honesty. When in a good mood, has a finely tuned and generally accurate sense of justice.<br>• Enjoys art and shows promise in this area.<br>• Is a loyal and dependable friend (though he has no friends because of his disturbing behavior). |
| 2. Identify his challenges | • Gets frustrated quickly and reacts out of proportion to the stressor.<br>• May refuse to follow instructions and gets argumentative with his teachers.<br>• When sad and depressed, may not ask for help.<br>• May misread the intentions of other kids in the class and believe people are out to get him when they are not.<br>• May not show understanding of the informal rules of play and social situations.<br>• May run away from school when he becomes agitated. |
| 3. Identify his current motivators | • Computer time.<br>• Points toward the new anime writing program he wants (parents are providing this incentive, school is keeping score).<br>• Praise for his work or just noticing and praising his accomplishments.<br>• Time with Mr. Jones, the school's computer manager, whom he greatly respects. |
| 4. Identify the best classroom environment | • The 14 essential characteristics for educating the AS-plus-BD child are implemented as appropriate.<br>• His class is highly structured, stimulating but predictable.<br>• Teachers are trained in rage de-escalation and are fluent in use of the sequenced interventions described in his behavior management plan.<br>• The child is able to move around the classroom as long as he has his mood and body under control.<br>• Other students understand the challenges faced by the AS-plus-BD child. They understand that many kids have similar issues, that nobody is perfect, and that the order of the day is tolerance and compassion. |
| 6. Identify staff behaviors that are part of the solution – keeping the child focused and following | • Note the behavior that is problematic and privately ask the child if you can do something to help.<br>• Use empathetic language to bridge and redirect, "Sean, you seem to be getting frustrated. How can I help?" Give him a choice that helps him deal with his frustration. Do not show anger, embarrass him in front of others, or demand compliance.<br>• Use redirection as needed. If agitation occurs because of a task requirement and he is not able to benefit from more explanation, ask him to complete a substitute activity. |
| 7. Identify staff behaviors that are part of the problem | • Inconsistent classroom rules or requirements; unpredictability.<br>• Ignoring buildup in the child's frustration level due to misunderstanding of the task or directions.<br>• Ignoring taunting by other students.<br>• Staff anger or threatening manner.<br>• Putting task demands on the child when he is experiencing challenges related to his diagnosis. |

## Key Aspects of a Behavior Management Plan for a 9-Year-Old Child with AS Plus BD with Features of Rage Dyscontrol (continued)

| | |
|---|---|
| 8. Identify action to be taken in the event of destabilization | • *Use a matter-of-fact verbal style that* normalizes the child's restlessness and does not put him down. |
| | • *Encourage use of the pass signal* through which a child may notify his teacher that he needs to go to the reflection/refuge area to self-calm. (part of the room set aside with music, earphones, reading, and drawing materials) |
| | • *Do not argue with him.* Let him have the last word and allow him to cool off. |
| | • *Use descriptive, behavioral language.* "You are swearing. When you show me that you can use other words to explain what is frustrating you, I will be glad to help you at the computer." Use choices. "When you have calmed down, would you like to work with your team or work by yourself on the computer?" |
| | • *Deliver a verbal prompt, direct to refuge.* "Tom, What is the rule?" If behavior persists, say, "Tom, you may go to your reflection area" or "Tom, please go to the reflection area, will you?" and "Let me know when you return so that I can help you get back to your work." |
| | • *If he cannot be managed in the classroom, redirect to counselor's office to cool off.* Move into the child's proximity and attempt to make eye contact. Say, "Jeremy, you have agreed that if you have too difficult a time keeping yourself under control, you will go to the (counselor's office), please do so now. The two of you can decide if you should call your mom to come and get you. I will be happy to have you return to class when you have better control of your body. You may have two minutes to get your things together if you'd like." |
| | • *Remind child of possible consequences.* If he remains in class, say, "Jeremy, I have asked you to go to (counselor's office) and you have not left yet. I am setting the timer, and if you do not leave in one minute, I will have to call campus security to escort you, and we will ask your parents to come and get you. Please do so now." |
| | • *If he does not leave at this point, return to a place where you have voice privacy and call a campus security officer to help remove him.* Campus security staff should receive periodic updates on how to communicate with and gain compliance from children with psychiatric issues such as BD and HFA and AS. Otherwise, these staff may make the situation worse by being too heavy-handed. In most cases, the child in need of intervention by security staff is destabilizing because he is experiencing intense frustration and emotional overload. Helping him calm his body and mind is more useful than violently encountering him as one would a street criminal. |
| | • *Conduct an event debriefing after things have quieted down.* Give the child an opportunity to assess what happened, to explain his actions and to plan ways to prevent the situation from setting out of hand again. His counselor, teacher, or other trusted caregiver at school should encourage reflective conversation around what can be done to prevent reoccurrence of rage at school in the future. |

5. **Consider a mix of public and private services.**

Given the difficulty in finding an appropriate placement for children with the AS-plus-BD diagnosis, it is often useful to put together an IEP that is delivered using a mix of public and private educational resources. The law governing IEPs makes clear that school districts are responsible for delivering services even if private placement is required.

Private placement will only be authorized if the district has attempted to remedy a problem identified in an IEP and has not been able to do so. There will be pressure from the district to place the child in self-contained, behavior-control, educational settings or special schools. These placements may be appropriate for some children but typically do not offer the educational quality found in the mainstream classroom. Therefore, it is important that parents decide if a placement is truly the "least restrictive environment" (the legal term) for their child. If it is not, and if the school district refuses to change the placement, parents have a right to legally challenge the decision.

Despite recent changes in the law that sets up the IEP process, parents still have a lot of advantages in the situation, and they should not refrain from challenging an inappropriate placement if need be. Under the law, if they prevail in the process, parents' legal expenses can be paid by the district.[72]

Getting on the issue early is important. An improved school setting will help the child stabilize herself as quickly as she can do so. With stability comes improvement in bipolar-related symptoms and a reduction in both emotional and financial costs for the child, her parents, and the school district. Here are some different ways to involve private resources in the child's educational program.

- The child attends private school on a full-time basis, either in a day or in boarding school setting. The law that governs the IEP law (i.e., IDEA) has been interpreted by the courts as authorizing district placement of children in a residential setting if this is necessary in order for the child to meet academic, social, and emotional milestones, and the appropriate educational services cannot be provided to the student within the district. This is an expensive option and would only be taken if a child could not be served in a therapeutic day school run by the district or provided privately within a reasonable distance from the child's home.

- The child is enrolled in one-to-one tutoring with a private contractor (or an itinerant teacher provided by the district to educate the student at home). This is referred to as "hospital homebound" in some districts, and is used when students have a medical illness or psychiatric/emotional disorder that prevents them from attending school full time for core subjects or attending school for classes in their special interest or for social contact.

- The child is home-schooled with specialized tutoring services provided by the district.

These types of services are typical of those provided to families with AS-plus-BD children by school districts in the United States. Many parents report that though the school district may promise to provide appropriate services, the devil is in the details. This is why some families choose to retain an educational attorney to keep an eye on their dealings with the school bureaucracy and advise them if necessary. Although there is some cost to recruiting an attorney up-front, this expense may be recouped many times over by the voice the professional gives parents with the district

## Conclusion: The Prognosis Is Splendid

The child with AS plus BD experiences severe dysinhibition of the emotional centers of his brain. His situation is made worse by his AS-related tendencies for obsessionality, high anxiety, black-and-white thinking and lack of common sense. Fortunately, the brain continues to grow and, as mentioned, toward the end of adolescence a growth spurt occurs in the frontal lobes of the brain, the seat of executive function and observer perspective.

It is common for parents of children to report that their kids had the most disturbing behavior in the late-elementary and middle school years. I have found that at age 11 or 12, most children with the diagnosis are experiencing hellish lives. But parents often report that once their child rounded the bend on high school and got through the powerful anxiety that comes with graduating, things settled down somewhat. Some parents have reported to me that once their kids hit late adolescence, they started taking more ownership of their issues. Their primary challenges revert to the presence of the diagnosis of AS, but they are getting through their days without the major mood shifts and emotional explosions that define BD in younger children and teens.

Some adolescents and young adults continue to be severely challenged, however. If substance use is involved, there is a greatly elevated risk that they will continue to experience symptoms of BD.

Bipolar researcher Dr. Kiki Chang suggests that[73] children who receive early diagnosis and medication have a good chance of enjoying remission of symptoms as they mature. It would appear that protecting the brain from wild instability during the time that it is growing might result in intact coping ability later on in life. My clinical experience has taught me that a child has a better chance of "surviving" if his medication is right, he has access to treatment, and his life is stable. Child poverty is the one force that attacks all three criteria for remission. Sadly, a child's economic status has a lot to do with his ability to survive growing up AS-plus-BD.

Nevertheless, I think there is good reason to be optimistic. Many of the parents who bring their children to me for counseling are themselves diagnosed with manic-depression. Though they report wounds, joys, and sorrows because of "being bipolar," they are most often leading normally successful and fulfilling lives. They have learned to respect the challenge of living with a hyperenergized emotional system and are managing.

In the myth of the *Spirit in the Bottle*, the genie is depicted as destructive unless contained by his bottle. Later he is released to do great good in the world. So it is with the genius or "genie" of children in the AS-plus-BD archetype. As youngsters, their inner power is great but their ability to control their lives is not. In order to grow up to put their gifts into the world, they need love and fair but very firm boundaries and consequences. Given the attention and respect that they deserve, their "genius within" will some day find realization in positive ways that will benefit the child (as adult) and may benefit us all![74]

# Endnotes

24. Purse, M., & Read, K. (2005). *Mary Kay Latourneau, Victim of bipolar disorder?* www.about.com.

25. Lynn, 2000.

26. Hirschfeld, R., Calabrese, J. R., Frye, M. A., Wagner, K. D., & Reed, M. (2003, May). Impact of bipolar depression compared to unipolar depression. *American Psychiatric Association, 4,* 5-13.

27. Akiskal, H. (1995, June). Developmental pathways to bipolarity: Are juvenile-onset depressions pre-bipolar? *Journal of the American Academy of Child and Adolescent Psychiatry, 34*(6), 754-763.

28. Papolos, D., & Papolos, J. (2000). *The bipolar child.* New York: Broadway Books.

29. Papolos & Papolos, 2000.

30. Remarks by Dr. Demitri Papolos during his keynote presentation at the Jean Paul Ohadi Conference on Children and Adolescents with Bipolar Disorders, December 1, 2000, Chicago.

31. Post, R. M. (Ed.). (1998, March). (A Clinical Update text box). Data from the first 200+ patients: Persons diagnosed with BD I, BD II, and BD NOS show a positive family history rate of 41% for manic-depressive illness. *Bipolar Network News, 4*(1), 1; Rice, J. (1987). The familial transmission of bipolar illness. *Archives of General Psychiatry, 44,* 441-447; Strober, M. (1992). Relevance of early age of onset in genetic studies of bipolar affective disorder. *Journal of the American Academy of Child and Adolescent Psychiatry, 31,* 606-610.

32. Kupka, D. (2003, Fall-Winter). Special report: Rapid cycling vs. non-rapid cycling bipolar disorder. *Bipolar Network News, 9*(2), 4; Kovacs, M., & Pollock, M.S.W. (1995, June). Bipolar disorder and comorbid conduct disorder in children and adolescence. *Journal of the American Academy of Child and Adolescent Psychiatry, 34*(6), 715-723.

33. Kraepelin, E. (1921). *Manic-depressive paranoia and insanity.* Manchester, NH: Ayer Co Pub. (English translation of the original German from the earlier eighth edition)

34. Papolos, 2000.

35. Young, R. C., Biggs, J. T., Ziegler, V. E., & Meyer, D. A. (1978). A rating scale for mania: Reliability, validity and sensitivity. *British Journal of Psychiatry, 199,* 429-435; Gracious, B. L., Youngstrom E. A., Findling R. L., & Calabrese, J. R. (2002, November). Discriminative validity of a parent version of the Young Mania Rating Scale. *Journal of the American Academy of Child and Adolescent Psychiatry, 41*(11), 1350-1359; Wagner, K. (June 2005). Treatment guidelines for pediatric bipolar disorder. *Psychiatric Times, 44;* Post, R. M. (Ed.). (1999, June). Early recognition and treatment of schizophrenia and bipolar disorder in children and adolescents. Presentations, NIMH Research Workshop, Bethesda, MD. *Bipolar Network News, 5*(2), 3.

36. Perry, W., & Braff, D. L. (1994). Information-processing deficits and thought disorder in schizophrenia. *The American Journal of Psychiatry, 151,* 363-367.

37. Papolos, D. (2000, January). The hole in the wall gang. *The Bipolar Child Newsletter, 2.* From www.bipolarchild.com; Hendren, R. (2004). New research findings in bipolar disorder and pervasive developmental disorder in youth. In *Recent breakthroughs in child and adolescent psychiatry.* Irvine, CA: CME Inc. pp. 43-70.

38. Akiskal, H. S. (1995, June). Developmental pathways to bipolarity: Are juvenile-onset depressions pre-bipolar? *Journal of the American Academy of Child and Adolescent Psychiatry, 34*(6), 754-763.

39. Papolos, 2000.

40. Popper, C. (1989, Summer). Diagnosing bipolar vs. ADHD. *Journal of the American Academy of Child and Adolescent Psychiatry, 5,* 6.

41. (June 1996). Fact Sheet Number PKT 00-0019. National Institute of Mental Health. Bipolar Disorder. Prepared with assistance of Hagop Akiskal, Senior Science Advisor, Office of the Director, NIMH. http://www.nih.gov

42. Geller, B., & Luby, J. (1997). Child and adolescent bipolar disorder: A review of the past 10 years. *Journal of the American Academy of Child and Adolescent Psychiatry, 36*(9), 1168-1176.

43. Greene, R. (1998). *The explosive child.* New York: Harper Collins.

44. Kruesi, M. (2005). Treatment of children with conduct disorder and aggression. In *What's new in child and adolescent psychiatry.* Irving, CA: CME Inc. p. 74.

45. Greene, 1998.

46. Wilens, T. (1999). *Straight talk about psychiatric medication for kids.* New York: Guilford. p.167.

47. Hendren, R. (2004). In this lecture transcript, Dr. Hendren details the decreased brain "executive function" he identifies in children who are diagnosed with both bipolar disorder and a PDD such as HFA or AS.

48. Pary, R. J., Levitas, A., & Hurley, A. (1999). Diagnosis of bipolar disorder in persons with developmental disabilities. *Mental Health Aspects of Developmental Disabilities, 2*(2), 37-49.

49. Wing, 1981.

50. Pickover, C. (1998). *Strange brains: The secret lives of eccentric scientists and madmen.* New York: Harper-Collins.

51. McClure, E., Pope, K., Hoberman, A. J., Pine, D. S., & Leibenluft, E. (2003, June). Facial expression recognition in adolescents with mood and anxiety disorders. *American Journal of Psychiatry, 160,* 1172-1174.

52. Hellander, M. (2005). *About pediatric bipolar disorder.* From the website: The Child and Adolescent Bipolar Foundation. www.http://BDkids.org; Wagner, K. (2004). Diagnosis and treatment of major depression and bipolar disorder in children and adolescents. In *Recent breakthroughs in child and adolescent psychiatry.* Irvine, CA: CME, Inc. pp. 135-162.

53. Kleinhans, N., Akshoomoff, N., & Delis, D. C. (2005). Executive functions in autism and Asperger's disorder: Flexibility, fluency, and inhibition. *Developmental Neuropsychology, 27*(3), 379-401.

54. Frazier, J. A., Doyle, R., Chiu, S., & Coyle, J. T. (2002, January). Treating a child with Asperger's Disorder and comorbid bipolar disorder. *American Journal of Psychiatry, 159,* 13-21; Chang, K. (2004). *Comprehensive treatment of children*

*and adolescents with bipolar disorder, A Workshop Syllabus for the Institute for the Advancement of Human Behavior.* Portola Valley, CA. Dr. Chang, a leading researcher in the area of pediatric BD, considers hypersexuality to be one of three identifying indicators of prepubertal bipolar disorder; the other two are hyperactivity and presence of a depressive episode.

55. Duerr, H. A. (Ed.). (2000, November). Comorbid bipolar illness and substance use disorders. *Bipolar Disorder and Impulsive Spectrum Letter, Psychiatric Times, 7.*

56. Goodwin, F., & Jamison, K. R. (1990). *Manic-depressive illness.* New York: Oxford University Press.

57. Geller, B., Zimerman, B., Williams, M., Bolhofner, K., Craney, J. L., Delbello, M. P., & Soutullo, C. A. (2000). Diagnostic characteristics of 93 cases of a prepubertal and early adolescent bipolar disorder phenotype by gender, puberty and comorbid attention deficit hyperactivity disorder. *Journal of Child and Adolescent Psychopharmacology, 10*(3), 157-164.

58. DeLong, R. et al. (1994, May). Psychiatric family history and neurological disease in autistic spectrum disorders. *Developmental Medicine and Child Neurology, 36*(5), 441-448.

59. Hartmann, T. (1993). *Attention deficit disorder, A different perception.* Grass Valley, CA: Underwood Books.

60. Pickover, 1998.

61. Pfadt, A., Korosh, W., & Wolfson, M. S. (2003, Jan-March). Charting bipolar disorder in people with developmental disabilities. *Mental Health Aspects of Developmental Disabilities, 6*(1), 1-10.

62. Lynn, 2000.

63. Simoneau, T. L., Miklowitz, D. J., Richards, J. A., Saleem, R., & George, E. L. (1999, November). Bipolar disorder and family communication: Effects of a psychoeducational treatment program. *Journal of Abnormal Psychology, 108*(4), 588; Frank, E. (1999, November). Importance of stability in prevention of relapse of patients with bipolar disorder. *Journal of Abnormal Psychology, 108*(4), 579-588; Johnson, S. L., Winett, C. A., Meyer, B., & Greenhouse, W. J. (1999, November). Social support and the course of bipolar disorder. *Journal of Abnormal Psychology, 108*(4), 558-567; Reilly-Harrington, N. A., Alloy, L. B., Fresco, D. M., & Whitehouse, W. G. (1999, November). Cognitive styles and life events interact to predict bipolar and unipolar symptomology. *Journal of Abnormal Psychology, 108*(4), 567-579.

64. Hellander, 2005; Wagner, 2004.

65. Lynn, 2000.

66. Buron, K. D., & Curtis, M. (2002). *The incredible 5-point scale.* Shawnee Mission, KS: Autism Asperger Publishing Company.

67. Siegel, D. (1999). *The developing mind: How relationships and the brain interact to shape who we are.* New York: Guilford Press. p. 36.

68. Koppelman, J. (2004, June). Children with mental disorders: Making sense of their needs and the systems that help them. *National Health Policy Forum Issue Brief, 799.*

69. Miklowitz-David, J., & Kim, E.Y. (2002). Childhood mania, attention deficit hyperactivity disorder and conduct disorder; A critical review of diagnostic dilemmas. *Bipolar-Disorders, 4*(4), 215-225.

70.   Leibenluft, E. (1996, May). Circadian rhythms factor in rapid-cycling bipolar disorder. *Psychiatric Times, 8,* 5; Glassman A. H. (1993). Cigarette smoking: Implications for psychiatric illness. *American Journal of Psychiatry, 150*(4), 546-553; Tsoh, J. Y., Humfleet, G. L., Muñoz, R. F., Reus, V. I., Hartz, D. T., & Hall, S. M. (2000, March). Development of major depression after treatment for smoking cessation. *American Journal of Psychiatry, 157,* 368-374; Swann, A. (2000, March). *Biology and treatment of impulsivity across and beyond bipolar disorder.* Lecture notes, Stevens Hospital, Edmonds, WA.

71.   (2006). Excerpted from the website of the Child and Adult Bipolar Foundation. http://www.bpkids.org.

72.   Silverstein, R. A. (2005). *User's guide to the 2004 IDEA reauthorization.* Consortium for Citizens with Disabilities. Available to download from www.c-c-d.org

73.   Hendren, 2000. pp. 42-76; Chang, 2004. pp. 80

74.   Lynn, J. (2005). *Genius! Nurturing the spirit of the wild, odd, and oppositional child,* London: Jessica Kingsley Publishers. p. 19. This is Joanne Barrie Lynn's rewrite of the Grimm *Brothers' The Spirit in the Bottle* based on a version contained in *Complete Brothers Grimm Fairy Tales.*

## Chapter Three

# Evoking the Genius of the Child Challenged by Asperger Syndrome Plus Nonverbal Learning Disability

I n 1982, Dr. Byron Rourke, a psychologist and researcher, wrote a book entitled *Nonverbal Learning Disabilities*, in which he described a type of learning disorder in children that looks a lot like AS. Rourke termed the pattern of behavior that he observed in some children nonverbal learning disability (NLD) to describe those who had difficulty learning in any way other than through words spoken to them. If you said something to them, they could understand and remember what you said. If you showed them a picture, they could not remember it. In fact, it was very difficult for them to solve any problem that was presented pictorially.[75]

According to Rourke, another common denominator of the personalities of children with NLD was their intolerance for novelty. They liked the familiar and became lost and anxious when confronted with unexpected or unfamiliar situations. Rourke also observed that these children had a difficult time understanding the nonverbal behavior of others. They tended to take things the wrong way, and to be erroneous in the motivation they attributed to others.

Rourke theorized that these symptoms were a result of dysfunction in the right hemisphere of the brain, the area that is tasked with evaluating visual-sensory input (such as the nonverbal behavior of others) and then attaching meaning to it. Research has shown that children with damage to the right hemisphere have severe difficulties interpreting nonverbal cues and assigning an order of severity to another's expression of emotion. To these kids, a mild look of disapproval may be interpreted as a thundering, shaming rebuke and be met with a full-fledged fight-or-flight reaction that may include screaming, cursing, and crying way out of proportion to the event. The right hemisphere also is the area of the brain that is used to pull divergent bits of information together to form hypotheses about what is going on. The child with an underfunctioning right brain has a difficult time doing this, and therefore has problems forming original concepts.

When the right hemisphere underfunctions, the left hemisphere takes up the slack. Its job is to classify, name, and memorize things. Rourke suggested that NLD children survive by using their excellent rote learning and rote memorization skills. On the other hand, their math and science skills tend to be poor because they demand a level of ability to manage complexity and abstraction that these children lack because of right-brain issues. He theorized that the NLD child's difficulty moving from specific math facts to formation of abstractions was the cause of poor math performance. He noted, however, that though the child with NLD typically shows cognitive delays around math in elementary school, she might master geometry later on in middle school and trigonometry in high school. These anomalies to his theory, Rourke theorized, are because geometry and trigonometry require memorization of theorems and principles and are less demanding in terms of open-ended problem solving.[76]

Another deficit Rourke tracked in this population was what is termed "motor apraxia," or the inability to plan muscle movements. This results in having difficulty with athletic activities that require rapid changes in posture and precise, rapid movement. Soccer may be out of the question, but a sport like baseball that moves slower and is more predictable might be perfectly okay. The NLD child's command of baseball statistics is unequaled and he will be able to gather points with the other kids based on this ability to talk baseball lore that goes back 30 years.

Because of their great difficulty in reading visual cues, coupled with their inability to learn in novel situations, NLD children tend to have problems making and keeping friends. They get frustrated easily, feel out of control a great deal of the time, and are given to temper tantrums well into their teens. Managing these behavioral challenges puts powerful stress on the NLD child's caregivers.

---

### Children with NLD-Type Challenges

1. Remember what they hear, not what they see.

2. Learn from what they hear, not what they see.

3. Have a difficult time handling novelty; they prefer the known to the unknown.

4. Have a very difficult time reading others' nonverbal behavior.

5. Have exceptional rote memory skills and large vocabularies.

6. Have great difficulty forming abstractions and solving problems creatively.

7. May have problems in science and math in elementary school because of requirement for complex problem solving.

8. Prefer sedentary work.

9. May be clumsy in terms of right-left coordination and movement planning.

---

## Assets of Children with Nonverbal Learning Disabilities

Faced with the gloom-and-doom tone of Rourke's study, one might surmise that there is little hope for children with NLD. However, taking a little different perspective, you will see that they have talents that can be the seed of success later in life. Here is a summary of assets I have identified in my client research with children who fit Rourke's definition for NLD. The resources that they possess may be used to construct strategies for life success.

- They have excellent verbal memories and are naturals for debate, acting, and subvocalizing memorized instructions for social behavior. While reading comprehension is a big problem, children with NLD may be taught reading strategies that can make this much less of a problem.

- They have superior ability to distinguish sounds and pick out tonal changes in people's voices.

- They are very good at solving problems with known variables such as logic problems and chess strategies. Once the NLD child learns an operation by rote, she may demonstrate extreme competence in its performance. Playing chess, for example, may be a favorite pastime because, although the game is complex, there are a set number of moves that can be made in any situation and once these moves are committed to memory, the child may be able to replicate them with great proficiency.

- They are highly organized and naturals as "rule tender"-type leaders, who tend to enjoy work that involves collecting, preserving, and classifying things. They are extremely purposeful and can be persistent in the pursuit of personal goals.

## Four Essential Differences Between AS and NLD as Stand-Alone Conditions

The challenges faced by children with AS may look a lot like those of children with NLD, including problems with high anxiety, sensitivity to stimulation, need for structure, lack of social skills, tendency for hypertalk, and postural clumsiness. Nevertheless, there are essential differences, and it is important to know these differences, when designing remedial strategies.

1. **Children with NLD have greater emotional capability.**
   Children diagnosed with NLD and AS have problems relating to people and are not good at social interactions that involve the give-and-take of opinions and preference, one of the features of what is termed "language pragmatics" by psychologists. Children who inhabit both neurotypes have a very difficult time interpreting the nonverbal behavior of others (and the verbal expression of emotional information).

   Despite these similarities, a more profound difference exists in the emotional lives of these children. Children with AS often have a fairly "flat" or restricted emotional range. They do not put much priority on emotions in their lives. On a 1-7 scale where "7" would indicate a powerful, compelling interest in some emotional state, they would typically score themselves as a "1" or "2." Children with NLD, on the other hand, tend to have rich, strong, inner emotional lives but have difficulty labeling and expressing their emotions. This problem, termed "alexi-thymia," is caused by damage to the structures in the right brain, which cross-compare words and their emotional meanings.

Children with NLD are capable of expressing a wide range of emotions. Parents of kids with NLD tell me that as challenging as their kids are because of their anxiety-driven temper problems, easy frustration, and cognitive rigidity, they have rich inner emotional lives and wisdom about what makes people tick. Unlike children with AS, they understand more about others' intentions (though they may not be able to read facial cues that signal an intention or motivation). Children with NLD, for example, may be extremely sensitive and open to important people in their lives, to include their mothers and best friends. They care deeply and suffer deeply if they think that they have done something to offend someone in their social network.

Children with AS have less of an understanding of the emotional domain and display fewer emotional responses with the exception of a passion for their work or special interest. AS kids are sometimes "harder to love" because of their inability to express emotion and failure to reciprocate emotional gestures. Parents of these children love and learn to relate to their AS children as rare gifts, but they may not get a lot of reward in terms of reciprocal expression of affection. Every now and then parents may get a sparkling moment in which their AS child expresses observer perspective about his life or achieves a breakthrough in his work.[77] These are precious moments that most "Aspie" parents learn to cherish.

2. **Children with AS are generally capable of thinking in both pictures and words.**

In my experience, children with AS are typically visual thinkers with huge vocabularies and well-developed writing skills. Whereas NLD children think in words, children with AS have a much greater capability to learn from what they see. The AS child has a preference for learning visually and may show the presence of what is called a central auditory processing learning disorder – he cannot take in and use spoken information efficiently.

The NLD child misdiagnosed as having AS may suffer greatly because of this misunderstanding on the part of her caregivers. Thinking she has AS, educators may set up a highly visual learning environment, which loses her completely. She needs to be told verbally what to do and needs a lot of repetition so that she can memorize the information. Most probably her rhythm of learning is the same as that of the child with AS. She learns best using the "three-step method": 1. give a concrete example, 2. explain a new concept with the example, and 3. provide another concrete example. Unlike the child with AS, however, she must receive these instructional stimuli verbally.

3. **Based on my counseling experience, most, not all, children with AS are better in math and science than are children with NLD.**
Both children with AS and those with NLD have challenges in forming abstractions. That is, it is difficult for them to learn from one situation and abstract what they have learned to another. But, in my observation, children with AS have an easier time with math than many other academic subjects.

I have tested this theory many times in my conversations with "Aspies" of all ages. One bright 25-year-old confirmed Dr. Allan Snyder's hypothesis that people with autism (and AS) use a kind of mental "abacus" that may be accurate even for very complex problems. Snyder's theory began with art, but he came to believe that all savant skills, whether in music, calculation, math, or spatial relationships, derive from a lightning-fast "processor" in the brain that divides things – time, space, or an object – into equal parts.[78]

Children with NLD do not seem to possess this kind of intuitive math skill, and they have great difficulty forming abstractions. The instructional delivery method in math is also part of the problem for NLD children. Math is generally taught very visually, on the board or overhead and in workbook format. Problems are drawn as a series of figures that are manipulated in such a way that one eventually comes to the correct answer. Children with NLD have great difficulty reading these pictographs and then putting the information together to generalize information to novel solutions.

By comparison, the child with AS may come to the correct conclusion, but his grades in the subject are often as low as those of the child with NLD because he cannot show his work – he gets to his answer with visual-intuitive strength but cannot break down the steps and sequences into linguistic number-letter terms.[79]

4.  **There are differences in the "genius" of AS and of NLD.**
    The genius of AS is found in the ability to study and understand systems and then devise ways of changing them. Whether it is a stream of water or electricity, or a complex mechanical system such as a ship, children with AS show a remarkable interest in getting to know the object of study at great depth.

    By comparison, the genius of NLD is found in a penchant for categorizing and remembering information and for making logical decisions based on this database. If the archetype of the AS child is the "Hermit," the bringer of wisdom, the archetype of the NLD child is the "Archivist," the consummate librarian, fact-checker, and information organizer and strategist. The genius of the AS-plus-NLD child will show the particular strengths of the Hermit-Archivist combination in the ability to remember information received in words and use this information to explore and change systems. The AS-related ability for white-hot focus on an object of interest is coupled with an extraordinarily powerful fund of information.

    There is potential for the expression of positive genius if the AS-plus-NLD child can learn ways to overcome the deficits in self-organization and social communication that usually come with his neurotype.

---

**Four Essential Differences Between AS and NLD in Children**

1.  Children with NLD have greater emotional capability.

2.  Children with AS are generally capable of thinking in both pictures and words.

3.  Most, not all, children with AS are typically better in math and science than are children with NLD.

4.  There are differences in the "genius" of AS and of NLD.

---

## Understanding the Specific Learning Disabilities of the AS-Plus-NLD Child

Research on the difference between AS and NLD indicates that children with AS can be powerful visual and auditory processors. Higher verbal IQ for children with AS simply means that this is an area of relative proficiency for them. Even though there may be a significant difference in their measured abilities to process auditory versus visual information (some AS kids are poorer visual processors), children with AS do not generally have a "nonverbal learning disability." The defining impairments in NLD lie in poor left-right brain hemisphere coordination, exclusive auditory thinking, inability to remember and process visual information, and poor abstract problem solving. If these features are present, the child diagnosed with autism or AS also qualifies for the diagnosis of NLD.[80]

Not surprisingly, the child with NLD will have difficulty performing the functions that are coordinated by the right brain hemisphere. Dr. Byron Rourke identifies the NLD child's most significant academic challenges as follows[81]:

- Difficulty with handwriting in early elementary school that often improves with practice and progress through middle school.

- Poor reading comprehension.

- Difficulty doing arithmetic calculations involving abstract reasoning and problem solving past the fifth grade. In later years, capability in math may improve. For example, the ability to do calculus and trigonometry, which are based on memorized facts (auditory memory is strength for kids with NLD), may improve.

  Despite Rourke's contention that geometry is easier for children with NLD, several colleagues who are special education teachers have asserted to me that geometry is more difficult for the NLD child they teach because of its demand for visual-spatial computation. These teachers suggest that the requirements of algebra and calculus for rote memorization give NLD kids an advantage. More research is needed in this area so that appropriate math education methods can be devised for children with NLD.

- Difficulty in science when abstract problem solving is required.

- Difficulty in sports and physical education classes that assume good right-left body coordination. The child with NLD shows poor right-left coordination manifested in challenges with any activity requiring coordination of the right and left brain hemispheres, such as riding a bike or tying his shoes.

Rourke also lists significant social-emotional challenges that cause more difficulty for kids with NLD than their academic problems:

- Poor adaptation to novel situations. The child has difficulty applying social learning from one context to another. There is an over-reliance on rote, prosaic, approaches to social challenges that may be inappropriate.

- Deficits in social perception (how one is viewed by others), social judgment (what is appropriate action in a certain situation), and interaction skills.

- Tendency toward internalization. Children with NLD keep their feelings inside and are subject to high anxiety and depression.

- Hyperactivity. The origin of this hyperactivity is most probably high anxiety – a frantic search to get their needs met in the absence of the ability to cope with the stress of their lives.

## Strategies for Evoking the Genius of the AS-Plus-NLD Neurotype at School

There is great potential for positive genius if the child can learn ways to overcome the deficits in self-organization and social communication that come with the AS-plus-NLD neurotype. Because these issues tend to sabotage the child's success at school, we offer the following 14 strategies for helping the NLD child in the classroom.

1. **Use educational assessment to identify a possible nonverbal learning disability.**
   A spread in the child's scores on the verbal IQ (VIQ) and performance

IQ (PIQ) subtests of the *Wechsler Scale of Intelligence for Children-Third Edition* (WISC-III) has often been interpreted as one of the signs of the presence of NLD. However, according to Rourke,[81] about 70% of kids with NLD do not have a big spread between verbal and nonverbal abilities. Moreover, the WISC-IV, the edition of the WISC in current use, does not include verbal and performance subtests.

- In terms of cognitive strength, children with NLD are distinctive in their usually superior scores in the auditory-perceptual areas. There is little evidence that NLD is the core cognitive impairment of Asperger Syndrome. About half the tested children showed signs of NLD (as indicated by verbal IQ scores more than 15 points over performance IQ scores). Fifty percent is a large percentage of the whole population, but the fact that so many individuals with AS do not show NLD argues against calling it the core cognitive challenge in AS. Again, we see NLD to be a condition with its own signature of impairments.[82]

- Compared to children with AS, the child with NLD is more likely to score high on spelling, word find, and reading speed. Children with autism (research studies typically group HFA and AS together under the term "autism") have been shown to have lower scores on comprehension, vocabulary, and arrangement (deficits that contribute to their difficulty doing writing assignments).

- Unlike the child with HFA and AS, the child with NLD will show markedly lower scores on measures of spatial analysis and visual problem solving.

- Unlike the child with HFA and AS, the child with NLD will have serious problems in math. Math is difficult for kids with HFA and AS because of their difficulty in lining up numbers on paper. However, if math is required by a special interest, they often do quite well at it. Not so for kids with NLD. Dr. Byron Rourke suggests that they will have problems with math from the fifth grade into adulthood. There is one exception, however: If problems are presented verbally, the child with NLD may be able to do quite well at them.[83]

- Children with AS and HFA tend to gravitate toward science and have strengths in the area of scientific analysis. Children with NLD typically have a difficult time with science because of the requirement for abstract reasoning.

- Children with HFA and AS are usually better coordinated. Because of right-brain impairment, children with NLD may have very poor right-left coordination. For example, they report grave difficulties learning to tie shoelaces and ride a bike.

- Similar to children with AS and HFA, the child with NLD will have difficulty with handwriting in early elementary school. Unlike children with AS and HFA, handwriting often improves with practice and progress through middle school, however.

- Similar to children with HFA, the child with NLD will show poor reading comprehension. Unlike the HFA child, however, he will demonstrate excellent rote memory of auditory material.

- Similar to the child with HFA and AS, the NLD child tends to have trouble adapting to new social situations and to rely excessively on rote approaches to social situations.

- Children with NLD will share the deficits in social perception (how one thinks he is viewed by others) and social judgment so typical of children with the AS or HFA neurotypes.

2. **Make sure the student is fluent in the basics before throwing abstract problems at her.**
   The child with AS plus NLD has a difficult time paying attention because she does not easily decode things that she sees and because her mental processing time is slowed. To overcome these impairments, pace all visual instruction with clear verbal explanation and opportunity for the child to talk about what she has learned.
   Nonverbal learning disability prevents the child from making educated guesses about material to arrive at competing hypotheses or creative solutions. The right brain is involved in this productive guesswork in its ability to call up possibilities and try them out until the solution fits the problem. However, the right frontal lobe of the child challenged

by AS and NLD is not fully utilized in the process, so the child experiences marked difficulties learning new material.

The rote-memory capability and structured information processing abilities of the child's left brain must be nurtured so that he develops proficiency in problem solving less dependent on right-brain input. Lacking the ability to make good guesses, the AS-plus-NLD child should be taught the basics of the subject matter to rote fluency.[84]

Fluency in a subject area means that the student can permanently remember and access the information reflexively, as in the case of somebody who has learned a language fluently. Children with NLD may do well in the elementary grades because educational approaches at this level use a lot of repetition and practice, but when the child hits sixth grade, the teachers' expectations change and he is now expected to generalize and begin applying what he has already learned to new material.

3. **Place the AS-plus-NLD child with teachers who know autism and AS.**
   The kind of teacher who is best for the child challenged by AS plus NLD is one who has experience working with children diagnosed with autism and AS. This person will not make assumptions about the child's ability to form abstractions or engage in complex social interaction. She will be logical and visual, and use very concrete language. She will also avoid using sarcasm and figures of speech.

   The best teacher will slow her delivery and give the child examples along with a lot of extra time to apply new information to case problems. If she is teaching beginning algebra, for example, she must test to make sure the student knows the basic math facts (what rules are used to write numbers in certain forms and what mathematical symbols mean) and math problem-solving processes (how you solve equations) before throwing problems at him. He must be fluent in these processes because he does not have the visual memory and right-brain solution-guessing ability to arrive at a solution by experimenting with the material.

   The best teacher for the AS-plus-NLD child will also have the skills to avoid power struggles, punishment, deliberate isolation, and threatening behavior because the child does not understand these rigid approaches. His problematic behavior is not intentional.

4.  **Place the child in a learning environment around good role models who can demonstrate the give-and-take of conversation.**
    Do not expect the child to understand the informal rules of communication. Very explicitly and verbally describe them: "Sean, when you stand this close to John (another student/teacher shows), you will notice that his face turns a bit red, his mouth tightens, and he breathes in through his nose rapidly. This means he is getting upset. When this happens, you need to move back three feet" (teacher demonstrates).

    Adult role models should talk their way through situations aloud in order to give the child a sense of their "inner speech." He needs this kind of modeling to learn how to self-question, self-monitor, and verbalize each step.

5.  **Review old material before introducing new.**
    Keep a close watch on the child to make sure she knows what she is doing. Do not assume she comprehends written material. Things must be carefully explained to her. At the beginning of each school day, go over everything she has learned previously. Two steps backward, three steps forward is a good rule of thumb. She has a very difficult time following sequences and problem solving, generally. Make sure she knows what the task will look like when it is finished.

    The "review before new" approach helps the AS-plus-NLD child to remember class content from week to week and day to day. While the child will eventually learn complex subject matter, it requires repetition of essential concepts and it takes more time. This is because it takes a while to "cut the path" between the brain's left hemisphere that remembers and categorizes data and the right hemisphere that comes to conclusions based on the data.

6.  **Teach everything with words, poems, songs, as well as pictures.**
    Children with AS-plus-NLD challenges do not understand the 65% of communication that is delivered nonverbally.[85] Teaching methods should be as auditory for the NLD side as they are visual for the AS side. Carefully talk through the lesson as it is being written on the board. Assign a study friend who can explain the lesson to the child. Use books on tape and other kinds of auditory input. Be careful not to

assume that because others respond well to visuals, the NLD child will do the same.

Use poems and rhymes to help the child learn and remember things. For example, to get him out on the bus in the morning, teach him to subvocalize: "Two, four, six, eight, grab my backpack and for the bus I wait!"

If he is nervous in a certain situation, ask him to remember a musical riff that he enjoys. Many young NLD children show a sophisticated enjoyment of music – many have high musical intelligence and can be taught to write music at an early age. Use musical modalities to get through to him, help him calm, and focus himself in stressful situations.

7. **Help the child deal with her difficulty learning from materials presented visually by following the three C's of Concrete example, Clear expectations, and Clear feedback.**

Use many hands-on examples that show how to apply what the child has learned previously to everyday situations. To teach a child with the AS-plus-NLD neurotype the scientific method of controlled experimentation; for example, teach her how to follow a recipe to make peach crisp. To teach her algebra, have her construct a chart that identifies the number of calories and grams in certain foods by protein, carbohydrate, and fat. Have her determine unknown values by constructing equations that build on the information given. To teach her about the psychology of selling things, help her to devise a plan to set up a garage sale for her family. To teach her how to be a conscious consumer, give her a method for analyzing TV commercials and have her keep a weekly record. Then build from these concrete examples to teach her how to generalize to other situations.

Directions must be very specific, such as "Please do this assignment in your workbook. When you are finished, you will have written all the answers below the problems on pages one, two, and three." This teacher does not say "OK. This is free study time. Take 20 minutes to go over some of the problems in your workbook. I'll be giving you a short quiz before the bell."

Clear, real-time feedback is also extremely important. If the child is working on something for 15 minutes, her work should be reviewed immediately with corrective suggestions and praise given soon after. The use of charting methods in which the student evaluates her own work with the help of the teacher is an excellent way to build toward fluency.

In a social setting, the AS-plus-NLD child should get feedback on her successes immediately. If she shows generosity or lessening of anxiety when it comes to turn-taking at an athletic event, for example, her coach is well advised to take her aside as soon as possible and praise her: "I know it's difficult for you to wait your turn when we're choosing teams, but you did great today! Keep up the good work." If she is less reactive at home, she should hear, "You know, Caitlin, this is the kind of situation (a disagreement over a chore) that would have driven you up the wall in the past. But I just saw you take a breath and compose yourself before you responded to me, and I appreciate your being calm!"

The AS-plus-NLD child needs to know exactly what you want her to do, how to measure when it is accomplished, and the positive consequence she will realize from the accomplishment.

8. **Teach the child how to *sense* his emotions.**
The primary challenge faced by the AS child with NLD challenges is in labeling his emotions and sorting them into categories. A neurotypical child is able to say to himself, "Now I'm feeling sad. Before I was feeling angry. I will get over this eventually." Because the NLD child's left-brain language centers may not communicate with his right-brain feeling centers, he has a difficult time sorting out his emotions and may feel painfully confused. He will freeze up in intensely emotional situations and get angry or cry.

I term this phenomenon the "grape in the throat" response, because the child will seem desperate to tell others what he is experiencing and at the same time be unable to sort things out and get the words out. To make the problem worse, his right brain does not decode others' nonverbal behavior, so he is at a loss in understanding what they are experiencing. Problems related to labeling emotions and decoding nonverbal material make the child look like he doesn't care about others, but this is not the case. He cares deeply but cannot express his caring.

To help the AS-plus-NLD child in situations like this, you must build on his analytic auditory strengths and facility for rote memory. Begin by getting his buy-in for some exercises to work on this issue.

- Teach the child to decode his emotional states by building body awareness. Ask the child to look in the mirror and tell you what his face looks like when he is experiencing a certain emotion. Pay attention to the discrete aspects of his face: "When I am angry, my eyes feel and look tight. My mouth looks tight and feels dry. When I am happy, I speak slowly, and my mouth turns upward in a smile position." Ask him to describe emotional situations and categorize where he feels sensations in his body. For example, "When I am afraid, my breath is shallow and I breathe from my upper chest" (demonstrate). Ask him, "When you are angry, what does the tone of your voice sound like? When do you feel this way?"

- Role-play with him to teach him how to recognize emotional states in others. Have him pay attention to the details of your look as you demonstrate emotions. "When I squint my eyes, I am angry. When my eyes are open wide, I may be frightened or surprised." Acknowledge his feelings of confusion and failure as he works on his emotional skill building. Acknowledge his effort and success as well.

- Teach him how to self-talk his way out of situations that provoke meltdown.

9. **Teach the child anger management.**

- Because of the psychological dynamics described above, the child with NLD is subject to frequent meltdowns. This situation is made worse at school where he is frequently the target of bullies. He needs anger-management skills. Here is a method for helping him use his innate gift for auditory memory to manage his anger.

A. Teach him how to sense when he is angry by using the body awareness suggestions noted earlier.

B. Then, teach him about the "anger triangle." That is, when someone gets angry, three things happen that can make the situation worse. First, his thoughts speed up and become less rational and more catastrophic: "I am in danger. I must defend myself. I hate this (other) person." Second, his body reacts; his heart rate speeds up, his jaws tighten, breath comes from the upper chest and is shallow; knees feel weak. Third, he does things, including anger actions, that worsen the situation, such as throwing over a desk at school or threatening others.

All three of these points on the triangle can develop synergistic interaction, each making the other worse. So the trick is to find ways to calm thoughts, body, and behavior. Each affects the other for better or worse.

**Anger Triangle**

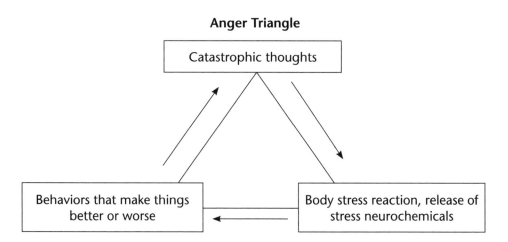

C. Pick a situation involving an emotional expression that causes the child problems. First, ask him what is happening in his body and mind when he experiences the situation. Then give him a script to subvocalize to himself to loosen up his anxiety. Finally, play the situation through until he feels more relaxed and confident.

Child:  "I can't stand it when my coach yells at me when I'm at bat" (in his school softball play).

Adult:  "What are you feeling in your body when this happens?"

Child:  "I feel like crying. I have difficulty breathing. I feel frustrated. I can't think."

Adult:  "This probably means that you feel scared, trapped, and stuck, and don't know what to do."

Child:  "Yes. Sometimes I just throw down the bat and walk away. I can't stand it when someone yells at me like that, especially the coach."

Adult: "O.K. You are doing great labeling the feeling you are experiencing. You can call that scared (because your breath is shallow) and angry (because you want to throw the bat down and walk away). Here is a way to handle this. Say to yourself: 'He yells at everyone. I am not the target. I can handle this.' Then remember to keep your eye on the ball. Let's practice." (Have the child stand up and assume the batting stance. Play the role of his coach, giving him some heat for his stance. Then have him vocalize and subvocalize his response.) "How did that feel to you?"

Child: "Better, but I'm still angry."

Adult: "Good. You are not scared any more. Make the anger work for you. Put it into your swing so that you power the ball so far into the outfield that you're guaranteed a run!"

**10. Build on the child's excellent verbal memory to help her succeed.** Help her remember what to do. The child with AS plus NLD benefits from analyzing challenging social situations and participating in devising solutions to a problem. However, she will become highly anxious in stressful situations and needs ways to remember how to behave more effectively. For example, a child may lose it and backtalk the substitute teacher who does not know the classroom routine and tries to enforce another schedule on her. The school needs to take the child's difficulty with novelty into consideration when trying to come up with a consequence for behavior. Procedures should be in place to help the child when anxiety develops around task accomplishment or a new situation that she cannot master.

Because NLD children have good verbal memories, they can benefit from learning social strategies by rote. Borrowing from assertiveness training, they might use the following structure to stand up for themselves when being bullied by another child who is insulting them in front of other kids. The following strategies were developed based on my clinical experiences.

The NLD child uses a script taught by caregivers around the acronym "**S**am's **N**anny **D**rives **S**low."

Sense your reaction to the other child's insulting remark.
*(Mad, glad, sad, scared, out of breath, heart thumping)*
*"OK. I've got the heart pounding, my head feels hot, and my breathing is shallow."*

Name the feeling you are experiencing: anxious, angry, etc.
*(Self-talk) "I'm getting anxious and pissed off at this little twerp and I want to punch him out."*

Describe the behavior of the other that is upsetting:
*"You are going on and on about your personal problem with me. I don't have time for this stuff."*

Specify the action desired:
*"I'm going to walk away and I need you to get off my butt. If you want to talk, I'm willing to talk too, but I'm not going to stand here and listen to this stuff."*

and

Breathe three times deeply.

Use of this strategy should be cleared with the child's teacher so that she can unobtrusively cue him to use it in the appropriate situation.

Children with AS plus NLD may also have difficulty knowing when to interrupt others' conversation. Because they do not have good visual perception, they need to listen for their moment to break in the way musicians listen for opportunities when doing a spontaneous riff playing with other musicians.

Use the acronym "**L**uke's **W**arm **C**lothing" to teach interruption skills.

**L**isten and track.

**W**ait for silence.

**C**ontribute on topic when silence occurs.

Conversational turn taking may be practiced casually at home or it may occur in a therapeutic setting. The NLD child needs a lot of help to overcome his inability to pick up nonverbal social cues.

**11. Use mechanical devices to compensate for mental processing difficulties.**

AS-plus-NLD children benefit from the use of hand-held electronic planners, unlike children challenged by AD/HD. After all, it is only natural for a child who inhabits the Archivist archetype to enjoy a state-of-the-art tool of the trade!

Because they learn from what they hear, AS-plus-NLD children should have access to books on tape for all coursework and should be provided with a calculator to bridge fundamental deficits in cognitive processing of math problems.

**12. Give the child practice in discerning visual details.**

Children with NLD have problems with visual discrimination – sorting out differences between things and identifying similarities. They also have problems sorting out and understanding their own emotional states. Therefore, it is important to provide opportunities for training the ability to discern the details of things more clearly.

- "How far from our house down the street is Max's house, in feet and meters?"

- "What do you notice about Mt. Rainier this morning? Are there clouds swirling around the summit?"

- "How do you feel on the first day of your job? Mad, frustrated, scared? Where do you feel frustrated in your body? Your eyes, your jaw, your gut?"

- "When reading, do you remember to ask yourself, 'Do I understand what I am reading or do I need to go back for more details from the beginning?'"

- "What do you think that look on Mr. Peterson's face meant when you told him off? Was he angry, scared, bored?"

**13. Encourage cross-patterned sports activities to remedy motor deficits.**

Clumsiness and cognitive deficits seen in the child with AS plus NLD are caused by poor coordination of the left and right hemispheres of the brain and the underfunctioning of the right hemisphere's ability to organize activity – both mental and physical.

Byron Rourke observed that NLD children prefer sedentary work.[86] I theorize that this preference for a sedentary lifestyle is a result of the high anxiety that children with NLD experience from dealing with novelty. Sports that require right and left body coordination improve the neural connections between brain hemispheres and work to heal the deficits associated with NLD. Encourage coordination sports such as swimming, skating, and skiing, or an appropriate martial art.

Many of my young clients with NLD, AS, and other neurotypes have greatly benefited from participation in the martial arts, Karate, Kendo (sword fighting), Aikido (precise movement), Judo, and Tai-kubuto (a combination approach). These practices teach identification of small movements and feelings, the importance of keeping composed under stress and, generally, a respect for authority. All of these learning outcomes are positive for children with NLD.

Caregivers do these kids a great service by putting athletic activities into their routines that require them to perform gracefully while strengthening their bodies. This kind of experience also strengthens the child's concept of himself as a physical being. He feels good about himself when he looks at himself in the mirror. Participation in a neurologically beneficial sport can teach the child self-control and motivation while the serotonergic effect of the exercise helps him keep his mood up.

**14. Help the child compensate for writing and drawing deficits.**
NLD-related visual deficits make it difficult for the child to do her work on paper. When possible, do not make her copy text. Use lined graph paper. Keep paper-and-pencil exercises to a minimum. Give the child dedicated access to a computer to complete written assignments. Do not expect her to produce the volume of written assignments that other kids are able to produce. Eliminate timed assignments.

## Conclusion: Recognize the Positive Effects of NLD on the Personality of the Child with AS

Children challenged by the AS-plus-NLD neurotype may be stronger learners and problem solvers because of the presence of both conditions. The AS child's weakened ability to participate in any social setting may be moderated by the remarkable rote-memory ability of his NLD so that it is easier for him to develop a repertoire of social responses. Further, the powerful auditory intelligence of the NLD aspect may give the child enjoyment of music or oratory. These skills in turn work to overcome the isolation he experiences from his AS-related introversion.

The fact that the child, by virtue of poor right-left brain communication, cannot think in pictures causes his nervous system to develop a powerful auditory intelligence. This powerful word-based IQ is the way the child's genius expresses itself.

Writing this, I am thinking of a recent counseling session with Ryan, a bright 10-year-old who showed features of both AS and NLD. My current focus was on helping him deal with a powerful anxiety state. I had spent a lot of the first session talking to the back of Ryan's head as he played with the toys in my office. He would not respond to anything that I said.

Finally, he turned to me and said, "Do you like John Denver's music? I do." I told him that I did enjoy the late singer's music. Then he proceeded to pull out a little pack of CDs and we put one on my player. Sitting on the floor Ryan told me that he would like me to draw pictures that expressed his feeling about each song. I happily got into the interaction, pleased that we were finally talking.

Looking back on the situation, I am moved by how resourceful Ryan was being given the limitations he experienced. Although his NLD prevented him from being much of an artist, and his fear of novelty made it difficult for him to just be in the room with me, sitting on the floor with me doing the drawing he could both enjoy the feeling of the music and see pictures in his mind of the scenes portrayed in the songs. This little exercise also complemented his AS side beautifully because it was indirect. Relating to me through the music, he was spared the stress of trying to communicate complex emotional experience – this was not his strong suit.

My clinical experience informs me that the best thing that I can do is approach a child like Ryan as if he were, in his young body, an old soul – the old, wise, obsessed, brilliant, hermit-librarian – and give him the respect due his archetypal status (without taking his curmudgeonly abuse). As I interact with him, I should not make assumptions about his motivation or "oppositionality."

The AS-plus-NLD child is hard to manage because he does not process information or solve problems efficiently. The challenge is to find his genius and communicate with it to help him bring his gifts to bear in his life so that he can learn to be more resourceful, independent, and successful.

## Endnotes

75. Rourke, B. P. (1989). *Nonverbal learning disabilities*. New York: Guilford Press.
76. Rourke, 1989. p. 98.
77. Schreier, H. (2001, September). Socially awkward children: Neurocognitive contributions. *Psychiatric Times, 17,* 9.
78. Fox, D. (2002, February). The inner savant (an overview of the work of Dr. Allan Snyder). *Discover, 23,* 2.
79. Rourke, 1989.
80. Cederlund, M., & Gilberg, C. (2004, October). One hundred males with Asperger Syndrome: A clinical study of background and associated factors. *Developmental Medicine and Child Neurology, 46*(10), 652-660.
81. Rourke, 1989. p. 80; www.nld-bprourke.ca
82. Cederlund & Gilberg, 2004. p. 652.
83. Forrest, B. (2004). The utility of math difficulties, internalized psychopathology, and visual-spatial deficits to identify children with the nonverbal learning disability syndrome: Evidence for a visual spatial disability. *Child Neuropsychology, 10*(2), 129-146.
84. Johnson, K. J., & Layng, T. V. J. (1992). Breaking the structuralist barrier: Literacy and numeracy with fluency. *American Psychologist, 47,* 1475-1490.
85. Argyle, M. (1988). *Bodily communication*, New York: Methuen & Co.
86. Rourke, 1989. p. 80.

Chapter Four

# Soul of the Scientist:
# Asperger Syndrome Plus Obsessive
# Compulsive Disorder

I n research conducted on matched groups to determine the severity of OCD symptoms, 50% of a group of people diagnosed with AS reported at least moderate impairment from obsessions and compulsions.[87]

Many of the children and adolescents who come to my practice with a primary diagnosis of AS say they are troubled by obsessions and compulsions. The following are some examples of OC symptoms in children that I have observed.

- A 10-year-old boy diagnosed with AS is wracked with guilt after eating a hamburger at McDonald's and must get down on his knees and pray for forgiveness from God.

- A 9-year-old boy with AS is unable to shower because he cannot stop thinking about the fact that he is putting his bare feet in the same place where his parents have put theirs. In order for him to use the bathtub, his parents must perform an elaborate cleaning ritual to "cleanse their body stickiness" from the tub.

- A 12-year-old boy diagnosed with AS must see four blue cars on his way to school, otherwise he will turn around and go home. He has established an obsessional fixation on cars in which blue cars mean "You will have good luck," yellow cars mean "You should be careful today," and red cars mean "Beware, something bad is going to happen." In his system, if he sees a red car, he must immediately see a blue car to balance it or he will incur bad luck.

- A 7-year-old girl with AS must line up all her stuffed animals in a certain order at night before she can go to sleep. She cannot report exactly why this is important except that "her mind" tells her that "something horrible" could happen during the night if her animals are not lined up from the most recent acquisition to the oldest one.

- Another child who claims that touching anything a girl touches in his classroom is dangerous reports that at midnight, all the "dangers" that have built up during the day are automatically "erased." He no longer feels "weighed down" by the "evil energy" he has accrued. Things are "back in balance." His OC punishes him for participating in classroom activities in which he cannot help but touch things that are forbidden by his obsessional introject.

An *obsession* is an intrusive thought that commands the child to perform some ritual or compulsion to avoid some harm. Children with AS typically experience obsessions and compulsions (OCs) but most cannot be properly diagnosed as suffering from OCD, a psychiatric condition in which the child's obsessions and compulsions are severe and chronic, resulting in total disability. When I compare children with AS plus OC to children with a stand-alone diagnosis of OCD, the obsessive symptoms of the latter are much more severe. In my experience, children with AS who have obsessions and compulsions are able to go to school, and they are able to talk about their obsessions with me. Typically, their obsessions change from time to time, and are treatable with the SSRI class of anti-depressant medication.

I have fewer juvenile clients with OCD as a stand-alone psychiatric diagnosis because many of these children are aversive to discussing (with me) the need to change. If they do come to therapy, they may be quietly terrified that they will catch something by touch, or that they will harm someone because of something they might do, such as look at the other person. People with OCD are dealing with issues close to those experienced by people who experience visual or auditory hallucinations. They may be profoundly disabled and distressed.

In AS, compulsions are often pushed by the obsessional feeling that everything needs to be "evened up" in some way to prevent something unnamed and terrifying from happening. In other words, the compulsion must be performed to accomplish balance, symmetry, and safety. Phobias, or irrational fears, accompany obsessions and further isolate the child. She may never go outside for fear that her presence will distract the drivers of cars in the street and therefore cause accidents. Alternatively, she may be deadly afraid of the germs that will "contaminate" her if she touches anything others have touched. She may feel genuine terror at the prospect of touching paper. As I noted earlier, an obsessing child may experience meltdown if she is not allowed to complete a compulsive behavior pushed by an obsession.

Obsessions and compulsions often accompany other behavioral challenges, including emotional volatility, depression, and hyperactivity. The child's obsessionality may emerge in early childhood and be pretty much a constant feature into the teen years.

## The Difference Between a Special Interest and a Compulsion

Many children with AS have special interests, and it is important to understand when a child is obsessing on something and when he is expressing his special interest. Typically, an obsession is marked by the thought that "If I do not obey this obsession, something horrible will happen." Although a child may fixate on his special interest, and be truly despondent if it were taken away from him, he would not experience terror in his loss. On the other hand, children and adults who obsess experience dread for their very lives if they do not obey the obsession. Also, unlike the profoundly agitating experience of obsessions, an AS child's involvement in his special interest usually calms and focuses him and does not cause him to become agitated or hyperactive.

Certain brain-based differences distinguish obsessional states from the exercise of a special interest. Performance of the special interest is a fixed and intense intellectual activity that does not show up on a brain scan as an irregular neurological activity. Obsessive-compulsive activity, on the other hand, has been seen with brain scans in the overactivity of the anterior cingulate gyrus, a structure that regulates our ability to put thoughts into proper sequences. This structure is rich in serotonin neurons, so drugs that raise serotonin in the brain have the effect of decreasing its hyperactivity and thus decreasing obsessionality.[88]

### Core Questions for Identifying the Presence of Obsessions and Compulsions in Children with AS

Detecting whether a child with AS also suffers from obsessions and compulsions is done by paying attention to the differences between the two states in observations of her behavior and interactions. Does she:

1.  **Appear severely distracted and inattentive, staring into space, when you know that she normally does not show this kind of behavior?** There is a distinct difference between the absent-minded manner of a child with AS (the "little professor" effect) and the manner of a child experiencing obsessions and compulsions.

    The child with OC shows a fixed gaze straight ahead. The child's eyes may flit somewhat to the right and left on the horizontal while she maintains this fixed gaze. Eye movement back and forth on the horizontal plane has been shown in research on how people think to indicate that they are "reading" auditory information in their minds – referencing thoughts as sentences. This eye movement pattern is an indication that the child is "reading" obsessional commands in her mind or performing some mind ritual to obey them.[89]

2.  **Become extremely upset, to the point of meltdown, when asked to pay attention?** Although children with AS articulate distress when required to break their hyperfocus on some activity, they are usually able to get over it quite quickly and move on. Children with OC articulate anger and a stubborn resistance to shifting focus and have a predilection to meltdown. In this regard it is important to differentiate melt-down caused by resistance to going through a transition from meltdown caused by a caregiver's demand that the child come out of his state of intense self-absorption.

3.  **Complain of not being able to sleep at night because of recurring "stupid thoughts" that she cannot get out of her mind?** Once the day is done, and a child's stream of distractions has abated, she is left in the uncomfortable place of being alone with her mind. If she is OC, this can be a distressful time. Sleep disturbance is not generally associated with AS so when it is present, it makes sense to inquire if hyperactive, anxiety-producing or bizarre mental imagery is keeping the child awake.

    Most children are willing to discuss these phenomena. Sleep-onset insomnia may also show presence of an anxiety disorder. (This phenomenon is discussed in Chapter Five.) In my counseling practice, I find it easy to differentiate OC from anxiety as a causative for sleep problems. I ask the child if the problem is the presence of "mind loops" or "gross thoughts he can't stop" (obsessions) or if he feels "afraid of the dark," "hears noises in the house," or is simply so "tense" he cannot relax. These expressions indicate the presence of an anxiety disorder.

4.  **Have a strong tendency to get locked into negative thoughts or is she unable to dissociate from the memory of some negative event?** Studies of children challenged by OC suggest that they possess an overactive cingulate gyrus, the structure in the limbic brain that governs our ability to put things in proper sequences.[89] They are constantly on the lookout for insult and injury and hold grudges. A grudge may be seen as an obsessional fixation on some injury that is perpetually being turned over in the mind.

    Many children challenged with AS have a tendency to black-and-white thinking and to be extremely judgmental, but they are usually able to drop a particular grievance once the facts are presented logically to them. Although irritable hyperfocus and grudge keeping are not primary signs that a child is experiencing obsessions (there may be many causes for this behavior), the presences of these issues suggest that OCs may also be present.

## The AS-Plus-OC Character Type and Scientific Genius

Many of the great inventors and scientists throughout history have shown features of AS with obsessional and compulsive features.[90] These eminent personages include Dr. John Nash (depicted in the movie *A Beautiful Mind*). Would Nash have given us his Nobel-winning mathematical models if he were not seized by his obsession for mathematical invention? Was the energy of the obsession necessary for this creative act?

Samuel Johnson, one of the foremost inventors and humorists of the 19th century (author of the *Dictionary of the English Language*), had to overcome a powerful OCD and incurable hypochondria. For example, he could not step through a doorway without performing a series of bizarre rituals.

Charles Darwin suffered from severe phobias, depression, and an anxiety disorder. Dr. Temple Grandin believes that his passion from boyhood for categorizing things shows the presence of a special interest and other features of AS.[91] Was he obsessive-compulsive? Probably the harm-avoidance anxiety he experienced is specific to OCD as is the thought that one has hurt others. Thus, Darwin was heartbroken that his ideas caused so much conflict in England and felt personally responsible for the upheaval caused by the theory of evolution.

Nikola Tesla, perhaps the greatest inventor in human history (as mentioned, he invented AC power and power transmission technology), was clearly obsessive-compulsive. He was obsessed with the number 3. When eating in a hotel, he could not enjoy his meal without first lifting each napkin and then discarding it to form a large pile on the table. After each dish arrived, he compulsively counted the number of items before eating. His life also showed features of AS and autism. He was singularly interested in scientific invention, had very poor social skills, strange sensory cravings, and savantic mathematical ability. In addition, he showed features of the "aloof" personality type for persons with autism that Dr. Lorna Wing has identified in her research. Clifford Pickover writes about Tesla in *Strange Brains:*

> Tesla looked at many facets of life in terms of invention. Humans were automatons, whom he called 'meat machines' responding like robots to their environment. People had no wills. Their acts were simply mechanical reactions to external stimuli.[92]

The lives of these luminaries suggest that it was their obsessionality that supplied the energy necessary to keep pressing for a solution to a problem when lesser souls had dropped away from the exploration exhausted from trips up blind alleys. The wisdom to draw from this brief look at brilliant-mindedness is that the genius that drives a child to accomplishment in his life also may cause him, and us as his caregivers, great suffering. The elementary school years are the most difficult in this regard, but with creativity and patience we will stay one step ahead of his obsessions and be strong enough to encounter them when necessary or let them go when that is the right thing to do.

### The Thin Line Between Obsessionality and Psychosis

In my practice, I work with children with AS who are also challenged by psychosis. Among my clients, this condition is not as common with these children as it is with children with HFA. When it occurs, the child will have delusions and bizarre beliefs such as weird conspiracy theories; she will think people are following her or watching her; her speech and movement will be agitated, jerky, and unpredictable; and she may talk nonsense or show severe distractibility and confusion. All of the absent-mindedness and social ineptitude that goes with her AS will be worse. In order for a person to "make sense" to himself and others, the thought process has to be a structure. In acute psychosis this structure disintegrates and the person stops making sense.

Obsessions and compulsions in children and teens with AS may take on a psychotic tone. It is important to know when the child is experiencing OCD and when he is psychotic. Different parenting, schooling, and treatment approaches are indicated depending on the proper diagnosis. The example of an AS child with a germ OCD illustrates the importance of making the distinction between OCD and psychosis. One child may have a simple germ obsession. He washes his hands 70 times a day. He is deeply offended by the sight of a strand of hair in the bathtub and he will not touch anything that (fill in the blank _____ his dad, his mom, any girl) has touched.

A child with this kind of obsession is "delusional" in the sense that his way of looking at the situation is not real; it is an illusion. But he is not psychotic. His parents are able to talk with him about the germ phobia. He may accept medication and agree to some limitations on expression of his

OCD required by his parents. At school, his teachers are successful with him if they do not challenge his need to obsess and work with his family (and their doctor) to get him stabilized medically.

Given the mix of services, this AS-plus-OCD child will get the opportunity to put his gift into the world, to express his genius. He may always be "anal retentive," hyper-anxious, and not the most fun to be around, but he will do just fine!

By contrast, if this child's germ phobia is expressed as a psychotic state, the child might begin to believe that his body is "infested" with germs that are eating him alive. He might begin to hallucinate. He might lock himself in the bathroom for hours, purging himself or washing his hands. And, he would not go to school for fear of contamination by other children.

Medical intervention would be the first order of business and the medication would more than likely be drawn from the neuroleptic (anti-psychotic) class of medications. Once the child's anguish lessened and his thinking stabilized, appropriate parenting and educational strategies could be employed to help him.

In my clinical experience, the most frequent error in diagnosis of AS children challenged by either OCD or psychosis is to miscalculate the severity of the situation. Children who should be considered psychotic are treated as if they are merely obsessive-compulsive. The antidepressants do not do an adequate job of helping them control the force of the obsession and may make the situation worse.

Misdiagnosis usually results in isolating the child. By high school, he is so far behind that graduation is out of the question, at least at age 18. Further, isolation increases the chance that the child will express his genius in negative ways, such as aggressive use of his computer online or participating in dangerous scientific experimentation without thought of the possible consequences.

Both psychosis and obsessionality are strongly heritable, so I look for the presence of each condition in the child's immediate and extended family and ancestors. If I see bipolar disorder or suicide, I inquire about it to determine if the person experienced psychotic thinking or behavior in the manic or depressed phase. Many children diagnosed as having AS with psychotic features experience mood cycling and, when their mood is at its extremes of mania or depression, evidence psychotic thinking.

I have noted that children with AS are vulnerable to instability and may express features of a psychotic state in their mid-teens. However, if the most disturbing features of the psychosis or OCD are treated, and the child is able to experience a modicum of stability in her life, the psychosis may resolve by the end of adolescence, leaving intact the primary AS. The adolescent will now demonstrate the ability to use more of an "observer perspective" in her life. This is most likely the result of a growth spurt in the frontal lobes of the brain that happens at this time as part of normal development. Thus, the "civilized" capacities of the brain have grown strong enough to offset the tendency toward chaos.

---

### The Difference Between Psychosis and OCD

*Consider the presence of psychosis if:*

- There is evidence of disordered thinking. The child with AS is unable to keep his thoughts straight and expresses illogical or bizarre ideas.

- The child acts agitated and jumpy in behavior and speech.

- The child is severely distractible and confused, to the point of being incapacitated.

- There is a history of psychosis, OCD, or BD in his family.

---

### *The Thin Line Between Sensory Integration Disorder and Obsessionality*

Children with AS are also vulnerable to sensory integration (SI) issues, and sometimes it is hard to tell the difference between an SI-related issue and an obsession. A child may refuse to brush his teeth, comb his hair, shower, or wear clothes because of the sensory agony he experiences. He is not obsessive-compulsive, but is experiencing severe distress that he may report as physical pain because of being exposed to certain stimuli.

To sort out the cause of the child's problematic behavior, speak with her about the problem and gently probe to see if she experiences obsessional thoughts around the aversion. If she does not, it is most probably an SI problem. Ask her: "If you are exposed to (X) will something dreadful happen?" If the child denies the presence of the obsessional demand, she is probably dealing with a sensory aversion.

---

**SI or OCD?**

When is refusal to eat certain things an aversion to the feel of them in the throat (SI) and when does it represent an OCD? "If you eat this, you contaminate yourself."

When is refusal to go to school an aversion to the lights, smells, and crowding of the building and when is it OCD- or OC-related?

---

It takes time and care to develop a relationship in which children with obsessions will speak about them. Go slowly, appreciating that the child's experience is horribly depressing and that helping her will require a lot of creativity and love.

## Strategies for Helping the Child with AS Who Is Challenged by Obsessions and Compulsions at Home

Devising ways to help a child with obsessions and compulsions is difficult in itself. Devising strategies to remedy the impact of OCs when AS also challenges the child is even more difficult because of the child's tendency to get lost in black-and-white thinking and anxiety.

The strategies listed here are designed to gain the child's ownership of his obsessions, strengthen his ability to deal with them, and prevent them from sabotaging his success at home and school. The guiding philosophy is to:

1. "name" the obsession

2. "claim" ownership of the problem

3. "aim" the mind's healing power at the obsession, not at obeying it.

This approach, called Response Exposure and Prevention (REP), is based on evidence from practice and research showing that obsessions and compulsions can be "de-programmed" by deliberately doing the behavior forbidden by the obsessive introject and then deliberately not doing the compulsion that would otherwise ordinarily follow the obsession.[93]

1. **Acknowledge the child's suffering; do not try to talk her out of it.**

   Obsessions originate within preverbal centers of the brain responsible for protecting the person from harm. This worry energy is powerfully compelling to the child, so do not dismiss it as silly or try to talk her out of it. She is suffering and will resist if feeling threatened. To gain rapport, approach the obsessionality with statements of gentle empathy, such as:

   "Looks like you're having a hard time getting to sleep. Are you O.K.?"

   "Looks like you're stuck in a 'worry loop' today. Is there anything that I can do to help?"

   Never shame your child for her obsessionality with statements like "Stop acting nuts! Keep it up and I'm going to send you away." "Stop that or you'll be grounded for a year!" Say, instead something like, "I am having a very hard time today with your obsessions and compulsions. I am really stressed out, but we will deal with this *together*."

2. **Use *natural response prevention* to nudge the child toward a reduction in obsessionality.**

   Behavioral psychologists treat obsessive and compulsive behavior with REP protocol. This approach requires that a child be coached through 6-8 weeks of daily practice in refusing a compulsion. Using this method, a child with a hand-washing compulsion would, under the encouragement of the OC coach, refuse to obey the compulsion. The two might stand by a sink after the child has deliberately touched something that sets off the hand-washing frenzy. Using REP, the child would refuse or delay for several minutes the urge to wash his hands.[94]

   Unfortunately, most children will not willingly go through the full REP process. It is too boring, negative, and stressful. Yet, there is good research evidence to suggest that resisting obsessional commands eventually extinguishes the obsession.

   I have always found it interesting why some kids "get over" obsessions. They will report dozens of obsessions that they have experienced, all now in the past. What causes obsessions to eventually wane in their intensity and hold on the child's psyche? Presumably, a natural REP effect is taking place and the obsessions are losing force because of it. That is, the cingulate gyrus is learning to calm itself with regard to a certain obsession. The natural REP comes about because the child cannot avoid all the things that set off his compulsions *and* he cannot always perform the compulsions because of social disapproval. If you are an adolescent boy with a hand-washing compulsion, you will have to "cool it" somewhat in front of your girlfriend's parents when you are at her house for dinner, for example. If her friends would be put off, you may also force yourself to resist the impulse to wash your hands around them. Eventually, the teen notices the hand-washing OC is gone.

Using natural REP, parents and caregivers manage daily events in a child's life to gently encourage the child to defy his obsessions:

- The child is encouraged to eat with friends because he cannot practice his dinner rituals at their houses.

- The child is encouraged to slow down performance of a compulsion or delay beginning the compulsion for several minutes.

- The child is gently exposed to worrisome stimuli for a short period each day. If he has an obsession about seeing bare toes and elbows, wear sandals when you go shopping. If he has a hand-washing compulsion, let him wash only once at the shopping center and then hurry him away for a treat.

- A good way to identify natural REP opportunities is to identify the environmental factors in place when they *do not* happen. For example, if they do not happen when he is with friends, increase his time with friends. If he is calm playing chess, encourage his participation in the chess club at school. If he is symptom-free during an outdoor challenge, sign him up for an "Outward Bound"-type of experience.

**3. Encourage the child to use his own mind-calming strategies.**
Your child probably has excellent creative resources for dealing with his obsessionality. To help him develop his own solutions you must be able to talk with him about his obsessions, and this requires a deep rapport. You gain this rapport by going slow and making yourself available as the child's consultant. If you are patient and he is suffering, at some point he may risk opening up to you.

This is an important opportunity to ask him if he would like help in dealing with his fears while keeping himself safe. It is important that any suggestions that you make not be construed as an attack on the part of the child that is running the obsessional pattern.

Take some time in your conversation to find out what images comfort him or give him a sense of strength and safety. Ask him straight out when was the last time that he felt really safe and peaceful. Keep searching until you have a set of images and experiences from his life or from other domains (favorite movies, role models, etc.) that seem to give him strength.

Now work with him creatively to select mental imagery that he can use to defend himself from intrusive thoughts. One kid might visualize a favorite "power animal" (for example, the kindly bear from the *Jungle Book*) who "eats" obsessive thoughts. Another child might imagine that he is listening to certain music that banishes fear and the obsession. Still another might choose to create a "sacred space" in her room, a place of meditation used only by her and to which she can go to relieve her mind of obsessive worry. In this space are crystals and other objects that "purify" the "negative energy" that she feels.

As a psychotherapist, I have found that if I trust the process of really listening and being there for a child with obsessions, eventually she will identify what she needs for healing, and it will probably be something that had never occurred to me. Practice patience, and you will be rewarded.

4. **Teach the child to turn down the intensity of her obsessive imagery.**
   When a child experiences obsessions, she engages in a mental process
   that consists of seeing the object of her obsession in her mind's eye,
   possibly paired with thoughts that contain the obsessive command:

   - Obsessing about germs, she imagines bugs crawling on her skin.

   - Obsessing about her personal safety, she imagines a hooded terror-
     ist sneaking into her house.

   - Obsessing about some insult from a classmate, she cannot get the
     other child's snarling face out of her mind.

   In order to decrease the power of the obsessional state, you need
   to turn down the intensity in the child's imagination. Here is a variation of an exercise I first described in *Survival Strategies for Parenting
   Children with Bipolar Disorder*.[95]

   The exercise is drawn from the repertoire of a type of psychotherapy called Neuro Linguistic Programming (NLP). NLP derives its
   effectiveness from the fact that it allows children to examine specifically how they look at things in their own minds and, by changing
   self-imaging, change performance reality. A child learns to behave resourcefully in a problem situation by bringing to mind a time when he
   was effective in a similar situation and by making the current internal
   image similar to the time when he was able to successfully deal with
   the challenge.[96] I have found NLP to be reliably useful in working with
   many types of neuropsychiatric issues in children because it does not
   require insight into the causes of a problem as much as simply a deter-
   mination to change one's mental imagery. These children seem to instinctively understand the relationship between perception, belief, and
   behavior.

**Turn Down the Intensity**

1. Ask the child a simple question about something in his immediate past, such as where or what he had for breakfast. Notice the direction of his eyes as he accesses the memory. Most people look down-left or up-left because this is where they store images of things in the past. If the child looks to the right in response to the question, know that he stores his memories of the past on the right side of his internal landscape. Once you know where he puts memory, proceed to the next step.

2. Ask the child to bring the focus of his obsession to mind front and center, at the 12 o'clock position on the analog clock face. Once he sees the image in his mind, ask him to rate its intensity on a 1-7 scale, with 1 representing a very mild obsessional state and 7 representing the most severe and distressing obsession.

3. Ask the child to "turn down" the light on the image, darkening it a bit. Then ask him to breathe down to his diaphragm to relax. Now ask him to reach out his left or right hand and "move" the (darkened) image to the place where he stores things from the past. Remember his answer to your question about the past so you know where to ask him to move the image. (It will be down-left if his eyes moved to the left or down-right if his eyes moved to the right.)

4. Once the child has placed the image in the appropriate position, ask him if this place for the image "feels" right. If it does not, ask him to simply place it where "memories might go."

5. Ask him to snap his fingers to "anchor" the image and let the internal imagery fade, returning to contact with you. Ask him now if the intensity of the image has changed. Many children indicate some change for the better, moving the image from a higher rating to one of more manageable dimensions.

6. Tell the child that he can use the technique himself whenever he is disturbed by the obsession and wants to lose it.

## 5. Minimize your involvement in the child's obsessions.

The general rules for parents should be: Minimize your involvement in your child's obsessionality, help her compensate as much as possible and get her into treatment immediately. If she is grossed out that adults have used the shower before her, work with her to clean it to her standards; do not do it for her. If she cannot eat a hamburger (although she loves hamburgers) without getting down on her knees to pray for forgiveness, do not take her to McDonald's. If she cannot tolerate the sight of her sister without having to do an obsessive ritual, do not require the sister to hide. Let your child know that although you feel her pain, you cannot and will not let her dominate your household with it. Expect an angry retort and let it go.

If her obsessionality is severe, get involved in treatment. Your child's issues are caused by an imbalance in brain chemistry. If she is willing to work with a behavioral therapist, she may be able to reduce the force of her obsessions without medication. Otherwise, the first order of business is to get a medical evaluation and recommendation for pharmacotherapy.

## Essential Strategies for Helping the AS-Plus-OC Child in the Classroom

Obsessions and compulsions sabotage a child's progress in school in a number of ways:

- They interfere with short-term memory and attention.

- They compel him to be impossibly perfect in every task.

- They destroy his relationships with other students in the class.

- They greatly aggravate his teacher.

- They push high anxiety and school refusal.

- Medication side effects may cause cognitive dulling, drowsiness, stomach upset, and other somatic issues that distract him from task accomplishment.[97]

These challenges are similar to those faced by children with AS as a stand-alone condition, and they are the seed of genius in the child. The brilliance of AS coupled with the ferocity of focus of the OCD character equips him in many fields, especially that of invention in the arts and sciences.

Your task as a teacher is to get this child through the curriculum and on to the next grade with her classmates. She is a child and her genius is untempered and untrained. It comes at you with raw fury. What to do?

Here are some time-tested strategies to help teachers manage each of these six OCD-related problems. The first caveat is that, as a teacher, *you cannot go it alone* if you have an AS-plus-OCD child in your classroom. Make sure that you have good communication with her parents and any treating professionals so that you can keep up with changes in her symptoms and medication. Ask these people how you can help.

Make sure that the child's OCD is thoroughly addressed in her IEP – both in the accommodations that are set up and in the educational assessment used to support the IEP. Obsessive-compulsive issues will sabotage the child's ability to reach academic and social milestones and must be considered justification for an IEP once the diagnosis has been made.

As mentioned in Chapter Two, I suggest that the child's IEP designate a staff member in the "guiding hand" role for the student. If her IEP coordinator has time, that person could provide this service. Otherwise, one of the school's counseling staff who has knowledge of AS might be asked to fill the role. (If any staff member has to work overtime to accomplish his regular job and work in the GH role, the staff person should be compensated. It is unfair and inefficient to put a resentful person in charge of a child capable of generating resentment from almost anyone that he meets).

1. **Participate in the child's healing by encouraging naturalistic response prevention at school.**
   Acknowledge the child's problems with obsessions and compulsions and identify as many of her OCs as possible. Don't give in to every obsession and encourage her to resist performing compulsions as much as possible. If, for example, she does not turn in classwork because it is never done well enough, require her to check it only twice and then turn it in.

   - Keeping track of success is an important part of deprogramming an obsessive-compulsive behavior, so ask the child to keep a tally of the number of times he had to check his work and give you that tally in log form on a weekly basis. Encourage him to continue to improve a little at a time. Work with his parents to come up with incentives at home and school to help him improve. In my experience, children with OC issues tend to be very diligent and scrupulous and do not lie about the progress they are making. If the child has a compulsive reading ritual, time his reading to make sure that he reads assigned material only twice, no more.

- Respecting the stress the child experiences in making transitions, try to keep him moving on tasks during the day. If his OCs keep him from being around certain children ("If I am around a kid in a wheelchair, I will get his disease."), work with him and his parents to gradually expose him to the stress of being around the "taboo" children. Eventually, he will catch on that nothing dreadful has happened as a result of violation of his obsessional introject.

- If parents report the child is obsessional about his homework and does not get to bed until very late, have him do his homework at school in a study-skills block.

- If he is perfectionist about handwriting assignments, write the use of an augmented writing device (AWD) or similar assistive technology, such as a laptop computer, into his IEP.

- Remember how painful it is for him to have an obsession and know that you increase his pain by preventing a compulsive response. There is a delicate balance to be struck between helping the child strengthen himself and not causing him so much distress that he cannot function. Talk to him about your desire to help and get him to buy into a certain amount of response prevention every day.

- Encourage him to come to you if he cannot stop working on a task. Just hearing the words "It's done and good work!" may give him sufficient permission to cease his compulsive redoing of his work.

2. **Help the child overcome short-term memory and attention problems.**

- Get in the habit of noticing if the child begins to space out or does not follow class discussions. At these times, give her extra slack for task accomplishment. Do not require her eyes front and center and don't tell her to stop obsessing. Talk with her privately when she is not "stuck" to figure out some "graceful exit" excuses that she and you can use to help her get out of the classroom without attracting peer attention.

- Think of one-to-one tutoring as you put together her IEP. The extreme distractibility of children challenged by AS plus OCD makes it likely that they will need to work individually with a tutor. This person should be both content knowledgeable and have experience working with children with AS.

- Allow more time for task completion and beware of machine-scored forms that require the child to fill in an answer circle. Children with OCD often need to get the mark done so perfectly that they will never complete the form. Have them circle the answer instead.

- Make sure that the educational assessment that supports the child's IEP gives you a good handle on the origin of her short-term memory and attention problems. These may be related to a learning disability, to a generalized anxiety condition, to the presence of AD/HD, or to OCs. Helping the AD/HD child succeed in the classroom may be as simple as moving her desk or allowing her to move around. Helping an anxious child may involve reducing some stressor in the environment. Helping a child with a learning disability may require one-to-one tutoring. Unlike these children, the child who suffers from OCs has a profound psychiatric condition. It is important to know what is going on.

- Designate a "refuge" where the child can go to express her OCs if they become unbearable. This may decrease the pressure she experiences from them and help her be more attentive in class upon her return.

3. **Help the child overcome social problems related to his AS-plus-OC neurotype.**

   If the student is ridiculed for rituals or obsessive fears, consider conducting a peer education program on OCD. The OC Foundation has a 45-minute film called *The Touching Tree* that may be appropriate for the class. Make sure to ask the child and his parents if he wants to be identified as a child with the issue. Some children appreciate others knowing about their OCs; others would be deeply ashamed if the word got out.[98]

- Look for social activities that the child enjoys so much that to participate in them he is willing to do battle with an OC. These may include sports, music, or field trips.

- Make sure that there is a designated staff member to help the child with social difficulties or to bridge to other children whom she may antagonize with her OC. Consider forming a group of children at the school with similar problems who can get together from time to time to support each other.

- Watch out for problems at lunchtime and make the child's refuge available if he cannot tolerate eating around other children or seeing them eat.

- Monitor medication issues closely. Know the side effects of the child's medications and work with his parents to reduce the impact on his performance at school. All the medications used to treat obsessive-compulsive issues, reduce anxiety, or manage psychosis have side effects that influence the child's performance in class.

- It is important that you, as the child's teacher, are aware of the child's medication-related challenges. The process begins by writing this authority into the child's IEP. (The school nurse should be part of the IEP team for any child who takes medication.)

- The most useful input about medication reaction will come from the child's parents. Children with OCD are exhausting to parents and because symptoms may be made worse or better by medication, parents tend to be keen and reliable observers. Use the wisdom they have to offer.

- Generally, the more severe the child's condition is along the continuum from mild AS, to AS plus OC, to AS plus psychosis, the greater the chance of encountering medication-related problems at school.

## Helping the AS-Plus-OCD Child Deal with Challenges of Medication in the Classroom[99]

| Symptom | Primary Medications Used | Side Effects | Typical Accommodations |
|---|---|---|---|
| Obsessions and compulsions, anxiety | Antidepressants | • Sleepiness<br>• Cognitive dulling<br>• Agitation<br>• Mania<br>• Hunger<br>• Loss of hunger, nausea | • Provide a signal system to leave classroom to rest.<br>• Put most difficult classes at beginning of day.<br>• Give extra time for test taking.<br>• Make protein-balanced snacks available. Having adequate protein on board facilitates concentration and mood stability. |
| Disordered thought | Antipsychotics | • Sleepiness<br>• Cognitive dulling<br>• Agitation<br>• Hunger<br>• Nausea<br>• Thirst<br>• Frequent urination<br>• Depersonalization[100]<br>• Weight gain | • All of the above.<br>• Make sure the school nurse and psychiatrist are part of IEP team.<br>• Allow use of washroom and water fountain on child's signal to teacher.<br>• Have a "guiding hand" in daily contact with the child. |
| Attention and memory problems | Stimulants | • Agitation at wear-off (rebound)<br>• Tendency to hyperfocus<br>• Appetite loss<br>• Increase in OCD | • Ensure staff is aware of the time the child experiences rebound so that this is taken into account when putting demands on the child.<br>• Have flexible lunch scheduling so that the child eats between dosing. |
| Panic | Antidepressants, anti-anxiety medication, and anticonvulsants. | • Cognitive dulling<br>• Weight gain (weight gain is associated with all the SSRIs except, for some people, Prozac and Wellbutrin) | • Make staff aware of these issues.<br>• Provide refuge area for child to regroup or lie down (if suffering panic attack).<br>• Allow extra time for test taking.<br>• Have a "guiding hand" in daily contact with the child. |

## Conclusion: Help the AS-Plus-OC Child Manage and Direct the Energy of Obsessive Fixation Without Experiencing the Terror and Dread of OCD

It is difficult to identify any breakthrough thinker in the sciences and arts who was not obsessive about his or her work. Looking at the situation this way, we see that a certain degree of obsessionality was perfect for the life of the luminaries who are mentioned in this chapter. Were these happy people? Some were reasonably happy, but most only seemed to enjoy deep happiness at the moments of breakthrough of their discoveries. This valuing of momentary joy does not conform to our cultural definition of happiness as contentment.

The heart of obsessionality is unnamed terror and dread. Is it unhealthy that it is this painful anxiety that drives a person toward great accomplishment? Is it healthy to live every day in the pursuit of some goal even if it means that a person throws everything and everyone else out of his life? Most of us would say "No. If the price of success is to live in dread of failure, I choose to live with neither." Everything should be in moderation.

Children who show features of the AS-plus-OCD temperament are not given to moderation, and their lives do not seem to be governed by the same norm of comfortable individualism that governs the lives of neurotypical children. The AS-plus-OC child *must* understand how the system works and will not give up until he gets it *right*. It is this fascination with systems that gives us pause to wonder if the genius, the guiding spirit, the soul, of this child knows that it must live in service to the larger system; to the world and culture. At some level, that sense of genius knows that this child will never live in the world of comfortable neurotypicality.

In the end, our job as this child's parents or teachers is to help him temper the extremes in his character to teach him to keep his perspective even though he may be tormented by obsessive urgency to reach his goals. We walk a thin line in this process between accepting some of his obsessions and not accepting others. This is an ongoing process in which we may take heart from the knowledge that, in keeping with the research we cite above about REP, refusal to obey the obsessive introject will eventually decrease its strength.[101]

# Endnotes

87.  Russell, A., Mataix-Cols, D., Anson, M. A., & Murphy, D. G. M. (2005). High prevalence of obsessions and compulsions in Asperger syndrome and high-functioning autism. *British Journal of Psychiatry, 186*, 525-528.

88.  Baxter, J. et al. (1992, September). Caudate glucose metabolic rate changes with both drug and behavior therapy for obsessive-compulsive disorder. *Archives of General Psychiatry*, 681-689.

89.  Friedlander, L., & Desrocher, M. (2006, January). Neuroimaging studies of obsessive-compulsive disorder in adults and children. *Clinical Psychology Review, 26(*1) 32-49.

90.  Pickover, 1998.

91.  Grandin, T. (2002). *Asperger's and self-esteem: Insight and hope through famous role models.* Arlington, TX: Future Horizons.

92.  Pickover, 1998. p. 36.

93.  Abramowitz, J. S., Whiteside, S. P., & Deacon, B. J. (2005). The effectiveness of treatment for pediatric obsessive-compulsive disorder; A meta-analysis. *Behavior Therapy, 36*, 55-63.

94.  Baxter, L. et al., 1992; Foa, E. B. et al. (2005). Randomized, placebo-controlled trial of exposure and ritual prevention, clomipramine, and their combination in the treatment of obsessive-compulsive disorder. *American Journal of Psychiatry, 162*(1), 151-61.

95.  Lynn, 2000.

96.  Andreas, C., & Andreas, S. (1989). *Heart of the mind.* Moab, UT: Real People Press.

97.  Packer, L. (2005). *OCD awareness exercise for teachers.* http://www.schoolbehavior.com/conditions_ocdawareness.htm.

98.  The OCD Foundation. (1993). *The touching tree: The story of a child with OCD.* Obtain a copy of the video by contacting the Foundation at (203) 401-2070 or on-line, http://ocdfoundation.org

99.  Wilens, 1998; Lynn, G. (1996). *Survival strategies for parenting your ADD child: Dealing with obsessions, compulsions, depression, explosive behavior, and rage.* Grass Valley, CA: Underwood Books.

100.  Depersonalization is the experience of feeling one is floating out of one's body. It is a profound and disturbing sense of numbness and inability to make contact with others.

101.  Baxter et al., 1992. p. 681.

# A Rigid Will, a Powerful Spirit: Asperger Syndrome Plus Oppositional Defiance Disorder

Oppositionality is part of nature's plan for self-protection during the developmental process. In order for the child to grow, she needs to differentiate herself from her parents and other adults in her life to form a solid base for future development. For example, a neurotypical child goes through a growth phase of "no saying" (the "terrible twos") that begins before age 2 and may go on for several years thereafter until the child feels strong enough about herself to begin allowing the "yes" word from time to time. The exercise of "no saying" helps the child develop a sense of who she is as a person apart from her parents. This is a requirement for the development of her personality.

Some children do not transition out of the reflexive oppositionality of their preschool days. They chronically refuse to comply with requests or directives from parents and only grudgingly comply at school. They do not do chores or homework, and even refuse to go to school. If pushed by a parent, they will have a meltdown. They do not listen to reason or show concern about positive or negative consequences of their actions.

Children with autism and AS are notoriously oppositional. I have seen examples of their strength and will many times. One such is the case of Bill, an adolescent I worked with in my practice around oppositionality. His parents told me that when Bill was 2 years old, they tried to get him to behave by threatening to deprive him of the use of a favorite toy. They said that Bill thought about their words for a moment and then went back to his room and began to bring out his toys one by one, giving them to his parents so that they would not be able to take them away as punishment.

My sense of the root cause of this oppositionality is the child's unique perceptual style. We discussed the "fixed-figure" perceptual approach of children with AS in Chapter One. This tendency to fixate on one aspect of the environment or one topic or one task, at the expense of seeing the relationship of this figure to everything else, shapes the personality and character of the child from an early age. And it makes his life hellish because it deprives him of the ability to have a flexible emotional response to others. Lacking this ability, he becomes a victim of every stimulus in his environment. To make matters worse, he may be ultra-sensitive to stimulation. This hypersensitivity makes him reactive to his parents way out of proportion to the real issues he is facing. The result is mild paranoia and the inability to see his own role in problems along with reflexive anger.

Oppositionality is not an *identifying* feature of AS or HFA because many children, including neurotypicals and those with ADD, show features of this kind of reflexive pushback. My experience as a counselor is that a majority of children with HFA and AS are oppositional. I believe that this is so because these kids tend to be highly anxious. I suggest that it is high anxiety, not "being AS," that is most often the cause of severe oppositionality. Corollary to this assumption is that management of a child's anxiety is the key to reducing his oppositionality.

## The Relationship Between Anxiety and Oppositionality

The child left in the "no-sayer" position has neither the practice in independent decision-making nor the self-esteem necessary to form a sense of herself. Current research tells us that having a coherent sense of self – a good answer to the questions "Who am I? Who are all these others?" and "What are we doing together?" – is essential for sound neurological development. Without this sense of self, the child feels like a nobody. As a result, she becomes highly anxious. [102]

Anxious children suffer greatly. They experience chronic dread that something bad is going to happen if they risk any new behavior. They tend to be so hypersensitive to stimulation that they experience the world as continually irritating, continually threatening. They are chronically on edge.

The Latin root for the word anxiety is "angere," the root of the word "anger." It also means "to be disturbed" and "to press tightly." This is a fitting description, as anxiety is often experienced as unbearable pressure in the mind, a dread of something unnamed and horrible, and it can show itself in the child's frantic anger. The body feelings that accompany the emotion are as unbearable as the mental distress: shallow breathing, nausea, trembling, sweating, rapid pulse, and dry mouth.

Anxious children are perfectionist worriers. They have trouble separating from their parents when the time comes for that transition. Children with these symptoms and behaviors often are given the DSM-IV diagnosis of generalized anxiety disorder (GAD). They are the ones who are afraid to go to school or have friends to their home for an over-nighter. Certain words upset them. They have germ obsessions.

Many anxious children express their anxiety by being chronically oppositional. Parents and teachers often believe that oppositional children are in "power struggles" with them – that they have organized a strategy for manipulating them. In reality, if anxiety is the cause of the oppositionality, the children are not motivated by a desire to gain power over caregivers. More accurately, they are motivated by a powerful anxiety related to their ineffectuality in the world. They feel like nobodies and lack the sense of "self-as-origin" necessary to proceed confidently and positively in life.

I noted in Chapter Two that Dr. Daniel Siegel's research on brain development and relationships shows that if a child does not have a coherent sense of self, he will have difficulty with "response flexibility." In practical terms, he will not know how to react to demands put on him and will therefore regress to his "default setting" from early childhood: "When in doubt, say 'No!'"

Dr. Siegel suggests that lack of communication between the right and left hemispheres of the brain may cause a lack of what he terms "mindsight," or the ability to understand another's perspective or intentions. This kind of "hard wiring" issue results in a lack of empathy and difficulty reading others' nonverbal meanings and regulating personal emotional states. A central feature of both AS and HFA is the lack of a theory of others' minds. This means that persons with AS or HFA do not "intuitively" understand others' motivations from observation of their actions, words, and nonverbal behavior.

This profound difference in communication ability is very isolating to persons with AS and HFA. Modern life is fast-paced. Efficient interpersonal communication is essential. Witness the speed with which neurotypical children work in teams in a classroom. Witness the efficiency of Starbucks workers as they move long lines of coffee addicts in and out of the store in minutes, or the amazing coordination it takes to negotiate a freeway cloverleaf at 60 mph. All of these situations involve minute, fast, and complex communication between people. If one cannot judge efficiently the motivation and intention of others in situations like these, life becomes very difficult. The result is that people with HFA or AS experience great anxiety – they are chronically stressed, afraid, living the "fight-or-flight" reaction on a daily basis.

---

### How High Anxiety Pushes Oppositionality

- The child's difficulty concentrating and irritability (GAD) push his tendencies to lose his temper and defy adults (ODD).
- His GAD-related problems with sleep and stomach upset contribute to his bad mood and make him more argumentative (ODD).
- His restlessness (GAD) makes him impatient and pushes him to annoy caregivers (ODD).
- His perfectionism (not part of the diagnosis but included in standard instruments for measuring high levels of anxiety)[103] makes it very difficult to come to reasonable solutions to problems.
- His muscle tension and (typically) sensory defensiveness (GAD) contribute to his bad mood and oppositionality.

---

Living the stress reaction in this way, the child does not have the opportunity to develop a repertoire of successful experiences with which she may identify. She lacks the personal autobiography needed for developing of a sense of who she is. The result of living the life position of "he-who-says-no" is that the child does not get to experience herself as independent of all the people she opposes. Her whole character is defined as "the kid who says no."[104]

## Counterwill

Dr. Gabor Maté, a person with ADD who has written a popular book on the subject entitled *Scattered*, builds on the thinking of Dr. Gordon Neufeld, a developmental psychologist from Vancouver, BC. Dr. Maté suggests that to decrease oppositionality, you build your relationship with the child and train him to make his own choices. Maté cites Neufield's research to coin a term for the type of oppositionality most often seen in children with ADD and other neurological diagnoses – "counterwill." Taking a line from Siegel's work, Maté suggests that it is not the presence of a strong will that makes kids oppositional but the lack of ability to have any will at all. So they substitute automatic pushback to any demand made on them. Education, not punishment, is called for to decrease oppositionality. The child becomes less oppositional as he learns ways to be less anxious and more present in his life.[105]

As a therapist working with an oppositional child, I have learned to put aside the child's records and diagnoses and try to enter into dialogue around her life and what she does to get her needs met. There is a reason why children do the things that they do, and that reason is not always immediately evident to adults. As the child tells her story, I learn, for example, how efficient oppositionality is in protecting her from the expectations of adults or how it shields the child from having to deal with the fact that she cannot meet the requirements others put on her.

Most oppositional children warm quickly to this type of dialogue. They are happy to have the opportunity to explain the phenomena associated with high anxiety, difficulty focusing, and counterwill. And they let out their personalities, sense of humor, and pain. My tone may be sarcastic, funny, confrontive, or encouraging. I try to speak in the language and cadence of the child herself regardless of diagnostic labels.

Across the board, there are common denominators of positive genius in most AS-plus-ODD youngsters. They are fiercely independent. They are courageous. Many show superior intelligence. Most have a compassionate side that is often expressed in nurturing younger kids or animals. In addition, they may have a powerful sense of personal *justice*. These qualities can be the seeds of the child's contribution to the world. They will grow to fruition if he can heal the powerful anxiety that is expressed in his oppositionality. Our task is to help him transcend his life position as reactive underdog, or chronic outlaw, so that his strength of character can emerge.

## Nine Strategies for Reducing Counterwill and Oppositionality

The guiding paradigm for reducing counterwill is to manage environmental stress: To the degree that we make the child's life less distressful, her oppositionality will decrease. This is much more effective than delivering lectures about the importance of personal responsibility or attempting to shape the child's behavior with logical consequences or punishment.

1.  **Build lots of calming rituals and routines into the child's life at home and at school.**
    A younger child, especially, might have "wrapup" time built into his getting-to-sleep ritual. He might benefit from having a place in his room called his "sacred space," "spiritual space," "altar," or "personal space," where he can put objects that represent people he loves and his positive aspirations. Let him know that if he starts getting upset about something, he might want to retire to his personal space with a cup of herbal tea and that you would be glad to bring that to him on polite request.

2.  **Adjust family routines to reduce stress on the child.**
    Because of sensory overload and difficulty with transitions, certain situations cause anxiety-producing stress. These include showering, brushing teeth, eating with the family, or being seen eating. Unexpected changes in the daily schedule also tend to unnerve the child. Consider making changes in family routines that reduce his stress but do not inconvenience other family members such as the following.

    *   Post his daily schedule on a large board where he cannot miss looking at it. Give him lots of up-front warning for any change and be prepared to give him choices so that he can have a say in how his day goes.

    *   If you want him to get off his X-Box and do a chore, work first to peacefully terminate his play on the game. Give him a sequence of warnings and ask for his attention to your request from time to time. If he does not finally comply, you may have to require him to turn

off the game. If this is necessary, empathize with his distress at having to stop. The act of talking with him gently breaks hyperfocus. Doing so too quickly can be painful to him and is experienced as someone actually yelling in his ear.

- For teeth-brushing hassles, get de-sensitizing toothpaste and let him pick out any toothbrush he prefers, using any of the technologies currently available. His dental hygiene is worth the extra expense, and the nightly battles will be greatly reduced.

- For dinnertime hassles, let him eat by himself if he finds it stressful to eat with the family. If the family does eat together, avoid provoking him by scolding him or asking, "So, how did school go today?" – the question that makes so many teens uptight. They simply cannot answer this question because an accurate answer would involve deliberately running the day through their minds and they hate to do this.

3. **Teach the child to monitor her state of anxious arousal.**

- Show her how to take her own pulse by pushing her index and forefinger together on the carotid artery pulse found near where her jawbone meets her skull on the left-hand side of her neck. Set up a minute-hand timer so she can measure how many beats occur in a minute. Children with AS tend to be excellent visualizers, so as the child takes her pulse, ask her to think of a calming scene and see if she can bring the pulse down. This gives the child a sense of control and reduces anxiety.

- Teach the child how to breathe for self-calming. Show him how to breathe down to his diaphragm so that his belly "sticks out like a balloon." Ask him to breathe in to a slow count of three, then hold, and then breathe out for a slow count of three. Physiologically, it is impossible to be anxious (therefore oppositional) when one is taking such a deep and relaxed breath from the base of the abdomen. Consider putting little blue dots (the kind you buy in office supply stores that are used to mark reports and files) up around the house. When he sees one, he is reminded, "Take a breath!"

4. **Limit the child's video game playing to no more than one hour a day.**
Brain scans of children playing video games show that while playing, their brains release dopamine in the same way that the use of nicotine or narcotics causes release of dopamine and pleasurable feelings. After prolonged video game play, dopamine levels go down and the brain becomes tired, less efficient, and given to irritable reactivity – similar to what cigarette addicts experience if they do not have a smoke. Once this occurs, doing "unpleasant" tasks such as homework and chores becomes much more difficult.[106]

5. **Try to see past the child's "obnoxious," oppositional exterior to the frightened person inside.**
An anxious child dreads feeling vulnerable. Operating from "fight" or "flight" programming, he has no way to sense if someone is friend or a foe, so he pushes back. Deep inside lives a very scared child. I have seen this repeatedly in my counseling office. A child may be scary, look hardened, talk like a little gangster, or savage his parent verbally, but inside he is a puppy. Parents and teachers who see through the crusty and insulting exterior of the oppositional child to his "inner child" essence are at a great advantage in terms of communicating with him.

6. **Start small, have fun, and build learning with positive reinforcement.**
The AS-plus-ODD child is easily overwhelmed, and this feeling brings out counterwill. To increase compliance help the child take control of things in her life. Start small.

- If she resists going to school, getting there three days out of the week is a big step. Praise her for making this schedule and work patiently on decreasing stress at school so that you can get her there at least four days a week.

- If she is shy and anxious about having friends over, just having one over for an hour to play video games may be all the social contact she can bear in a week.

- If she is wrestling with AS-related learning disabilities, when doing homework, let her work at it for only 15 minutes. Once she is comfortable with 15 minutes, suggest that she try to stay in place for 20 minutes. Too much too soon will stress her out and shut her down. The anxious child needs to be reminded about how resourceful she can be. If parents forget to note the good things, she has a tendency to forget or ignore these positive qualities and, therefore, does not have access to them to form a positive self-concept.

7. **At home and at school, create situations in the child's life in which he is likely to be successful.**
   This will help him pull on his own resources to manage the anxiety. If an AS-plus-ODD eighth-grader tends to have a meltdown when socially stressed at school, make sure that staff know how to calm the situation with empathetic listening and therapeutic respite from the stressor. Or give the child a job in the school library or on the school yearbook in which he can participate in the community without being the center of any social event.

8. **Help your AS-plus-ODD child loosen the grip of his fixed-focus perceptual style.**
   AS-plus-ODD children have difficulty getting unstuck from the object of their intense concentration, and benefit from practice shuttling from internal experience to external experience at the same time or among different sensory modalities. The following are some ways to help the child do this.

   - Draw the child's attention to things around him that he may find interesting or to sensations such as heat, cold, the smells of flowers, or other sensory phenomena.

   - Have him listen to music and draw a picture or write a mathematical equation that captures his feeling for the music.

   - Involve him in acting lessons or a drama class so that he learns to focus on the requirements of his part as well as to interact with others in the play.

   - Involve him in any kind of activity that requires movement and performance such as martial arts, dance, or athletic activities.

Children with AS often take a very long time to learn physical routines but with enough practice they will, and their powerful visual-kinesthetic sense can contribute to an outstanding performance.

9. **Try to reduce counterwill-producing environmental stress at school.**

- Keep in mind that the child may experience stress from crowding, the touch of other children, or riding the school bus. Set up her school day so that accommodations are made to reduce the amount of time she spends in large classes and other noisy environments.

- Being required to do tasks that she cannot perform or becoming the butt of jokes are both highly stressful events. Pay close attention to her learning disabilities and make sure that testing identifies her LDs clearly and that appropriate services support her IEP. Attend to the quality of the school's bullying prevention program to make sure these stressors from bullying do not push her into meltdown or school avoidance.

## Eleven Strategies for Building the Kind of Relationships That Bring out the Best in the AS-Plus-ODD Child at Home and at School

Research shows that bonding with parents and attunement to them (quality time) is essential for developing the neurological circuits (the orbitofrontal cortex) involving attention, perception, and memory – those responsible for "observer perspective."[107]

Building the child's relationship with significant others in her life is a basic strategy for building her long-term resourcefulness and sense of self, and ultimately decreasing her counterwill. The following are suggestions for how to do this.

1. **Listen to the child.**
   In order to find the strength within herself to change, the anxious child needs someone to listen to her issues. She will only hear her parents after she is assured that *they* have heard her. Use your time with her

to do the detective work necessary to decode her anxious reaction – to locate its cause and to plan ways to change her situation so that she has more control over her life.

2. **Don't get into power struggles and keep expectations clear.**
   AS-plus-ODD children benefit from firm, non-punitive boundaries on their behavior at home and at school. They need to know the rules and learn best in structured, predictable, and interesting environments. If an anxious child gets his back up about some demand from an adult caregiver, he will try to get into a power struggle because he knows this struggle – it has a comfortable familiarity to him and it gives him a sense of focus. The most successful parents and teachers draw the line on prohibited behavior while helping the child focus on his issues and verbalize them.

3. **Don't try to set the child straight on the first expression of his defiance and oppositionality.**
   Listen with your heart and let your feelings inform you of what is going on. Tap yourself on your sternum (the bone in the center of the chest a bit to the right and over your heart) to bring your awareness to the part of you that responds with love and concern. Listen to the feelings that come up from this place as you listen to the child.

4. **Remember that sometimes the best way to resolve a power struggle is to let the child have her way.**
   This option is appropriate: (a) If the issue does not involve the child's health and safety; and (b) If the child is incapable of meeting some demand you put on her. For example, you may:

   - Let her have a messy room as long as she keeps the door shut.

   - Let her read herself to sleep at night; do not insist on a lights-out time.

   - Let her eat by herself or have a say in the kind of food that she eats.

   - Give her a lot of leeway in doing her homework and let her take the consequences.

- Give her a say in her medication regime. Make it a priority to educate yourself and her about the range of medications used to treat her particular challenges. Working with your doctor, help the child choose the medication that best fits her symptoms that has the least degree of side effects.

Eventually, the child will have to start making her own decisions. You make the power struggle worse by thinking you have to prevail in any dispute. If a task is part of a child's responsibility as a family member, such as keeping her mess out of the common area, walking her dog, and so on, parents have a right to insist that she accomplish the task. But if a requirement involves the child's personal affairs or consent (such as her participation in putting together her IEP for school), it is O.K. to negotiate.

Some parents dig in and make a major issue out of every demand for compliance, concerned that if they do not, the child will get more and more rebellious. My experience as a counselor has taught me that letting a child have her way from time to time does not encourage her to lose respect for her parents or disobey them. In fact, the reverse is true. When it comes to easing counterwill, letting her do it her way from time to time tells her that you are in her corner. Of course, this does not mean that you let her have her way all the time or spoil her. It means that you look at situations on a case-by-case basis.

5. **Remember that punishment does not work.**
   The idea that behavior is changed by punishment is a fallacy when it comes to dealing with an anxious child. Fear of punishment makes anxiety worse and it attacks the child's sense of self-worth.

6. **Walk with the child two or three times a week.**
   Develop a familiar route and engage him in the walk even though he may complain a bit. Build your connection this way. You do not have to say a thing!

7. **Redirect as much as possible and avoid use of the word "don't."**
   Go around the child's oppositionality by painting a picture with positive language of where you want him to go. For example, do not say,

"Stop yelling at me this minute!" Say, "I'll start again when I know that you are with me." Or (using a verbal prompt to overcome short-term memory problems), "When you can show me that you are with me, I'll be glad to resume our activity."

8. **Pour on your empathy when the child is frustrated about something.**

   If he is having a meltdown because he cannot watch his favorite TV program, empathize with him: "I understand something of how you feel. You wanted to watch that program and now you do not get to. I can see you are disappointed. I want you to know that the tube will go on as soon as you finish your math homework. Can I help with that?"

9. **Know that the anxious child is visually and auditorily cued to your behavior.**

   If you are upset, the child will be upset. If you are calm, she is calm. Children with AS and autism have a difficult time editing their responses to stress. They tend to behave instinctively and imitate the emotional states of people around them. Be aware of this phenomenon when you are interacting with the child and give yourself time and space to take a breath, count to 10, and calm yourself down before encountering her about some issue that may be stressful. You will notice that if you are calm there is a much greater chance that she will remain so.

10. **Teach the child to verbalize his anxiety.**

    A violent behavior such as throwing over a desk or attacking an adult may be a substitute for the child's inability to verbalize frustration. Encourage verbalization and teach the child to use "shorthand" if he has problems expressing his anger verbally. Agree on a scale that expresses his sense of angry tension, in which "1" is a state of calm and "7" is equivalent to totally losing control. Ask the child where he is on the scale. When you get a number higher than "3," consult with him to discover ways to make things a little better – to move his internal stage to a "2." Remember that things that have happened to the child that you are not aware of often cause anxiety. For example, the explosion in math class may have been caused by the humiliation the child suffered in P.E. two hours before. Work with him to draw out these stressors and get him to talk about them.

When an oppositional child goes into meltdown, skilled management of the situation can yield very positive results, but often adults become reactive and lose their own tempers. Cultivate an attitude of cool observation of the stressors the child is experiencing so that you are able to quickly defuse tension.

**11. Manage meltdown.**

Here are some of the things the most resourceful parents in my practice do to be more proactive in managing meltdowns of their oppositional children.

- Get on the situation early. If you notice a look of distress on his face, see him attempting to hide or avoid stimulation, or hear the emergence of whining or "silly talk," he may be signaling that he is getting anxious and overstressed. This is not the time to put any demand on him. It is time to help him reduce the stressors in his environment.

- Give her time to move through stressful events and do not ignore nonverbal cues of stress and overload. Talk about the changes she will be going through in terms of what you will be doing. Give her a mental picture so that she can gradually adjust.

- Give him notice before desired transitions: Indicate to him, "I'm setting the timer now. When it goes off, I want you to put your shoes on. Then I will check in with you for next steps. After you finish watching your program on TV, I want you to sit down and do some homework. I will help you with it and give you a five-minute warning to help you prepare."

- In calm times, evaluate the origin of his meltdowns. You can help him get his needs met more efficiently if you know what is going on with him. If he is experiencing a meltdown because you have interrupted an obsession (and he must go back to the beginning to complete the loop), you may want to either restate your request at another time or get medical help for his obsessional condition. If he melts down because he feels overwhelmed by some demand you have put on him, you may want to consider the presence of a learning disability or some other cognitive or perceptual block to his ability to perform the task.

- Ask yourself what the best thing is to reduce the child's anxiety and *do that thing*. If she is frustrated at not being able to complete a task, try to gently redirect her to something else for a few moments. If she is carrying stress from a hard day at school, give her a chance to decompress. One AS-plus-ODD girl I spoke with told me that she needed time to cry and scream for a few minutes when she came home after school, because holding herself together in the highly stimulating school environment built up pressure that needs to be discharged. Her parents helped her by giving her private space and time to discharge this energy without scolding her.

- Rarely is it appropriate to physically restrain a child who is having a meltdown. Children experience restraint as physical assault and are deeply insulted by having to experience it. In terms of the counterwill model, the implications of this fact are clear: Decreasing counterwill is about building relationships, and if a child feels that he is under physical assault by his parents, it is much more difficult to achieve the rapport necessary for healing.

## Conclusion: Help the Child Manage the Fierce Energy of Oppositionality so That He Stays Connected with His Community

How you handle counterwill and anxiety in the AS-plus-ODD child's life has a lot to do with how his strong, often fiery temperament expresses itself. With the right home and school management approach, the powerful will of the child can be transformed from a destructive to a productive influence. The time and energy that the child previously put into fighting anything or anybody that tried to regulate his behavior is redirected to his own goals. He may still be stubborn, loud, and insistent on getting his way, but he remains in communication with caregivers and is able to control himself a bit. Later on in life, the qualities that now show up as counterwill may be transformed into a sense of "resolve," "strength," and "dedication." Our challenge as caregivers is to keep that potential future in our minds and hearts as we work patiently to teach the guiding spirit of the child's genius that he is not the only sentient being in the world.

We must always help the child see his connection to his community. Despite his exhausting behavior, we are best served by deliberately building positive relationships in the child's life wherever possible. Dr. Siegel's research shows that the affection and positive regard given to a child enables development of the circuits in his brain, centered on the orbitofrontal cortex, that enable him to see others' points of view and deal with frustration resourcefully. This research makes clear that it is not stern discipline that imparts the ability to go with the flow and be cooperative. Instead, it is the development, over the long term, of the ability to make and keep positive relationships and know how to make good choices. Showing positive regard in the context of firm and fair parenting is the key to overcoming oppositionality and nurturing the gifts of the child.

> This right orbitofrontal region serves the vital integrative function of coordinating social communication, empathic attunement, emotional regulation, registration of bodily state, stimulus appraisal (the establishment of value and meaning of representations), and the autonoetic consciousness. These exciting convergent findings suggest a preliminary view of how early emotional relationships shape self knowledge and the capacity to integrate a coherent state of mind with respect to attachment.[108]

Thus, we see that reduction in oppositionality is a matter of teaching the child with AS how to have positive relationships in the world. As we do this, through our example and action, we give him the opportunity to "wire around" his natural tendency to be stuck on little things, to rise above the situation a bit, to be a little calmer and a little more resourceful. Dr. Siegel's research would suggest that these outward signs of adjustment to life are mirrored by positive and permanent changes in the attentional system of the child's brain.

# Endnotes

102. Siegel, 1999. p. 21.
103. *Multidimensional Anxiety Scale for Children.* (1997). Toronto, Canada: Multi-Health Systems.
104. Siegel, 1999. p. 142.
105. Maté, G. (1999). *Scattered.* New York: Plume. pp. 72-74.
106. Amen, D. (2001). *Healing ADD.* New York: Berkley Books. pp. 29-30.
107. Sabbagh, M. (2004, June). Understanding orbitofrontal contributions to theory-of-mind reasoning: Implications for autism. *Brain and Cognition, 55*(1), 209-215; Schore, A. (2000, April). Attachment and the regulation of the right brain. *Attachment and Human Development, 2*(1), 23-47.
108. Siegel, 1999. p. 97.

# Part II

Assessing the Differences Between Asperger Syndrome and High-Functioning Autism, Tourette's Syndrome, and Attention Deficit Disorder

Chapter Six

# Strategies for Identifying and Helping Children with Asperger Syndrome or High-Functioning Autism

There is controversy among parents and professionals about the relationship between autism and Asperger Syndrome. Some maintain that AS is simply a type of very high-functioning autism (HFA). Others believe that AS and autism are different conditions. It is important to know the differences and similarities between these two conditions if you are to help your child. I feel strongly that, no matter how the two conditions are defined, they pose qualitatively different challenges to the child and his parents.

The pattern of thinking we call autism was first written about by Dr. Leo Kanner in 1943. Kanner, who was head of the Department of the Psychiatric Clinic of Johns Hopkins University, provided an accurate and detailed description of the characteristics of children we would now classify as "lower-functioning" autistic. All of the children in his study population were intellectually delayed and, if the IQ scales we use today had been available in his time, would have scored less than 70, the threshold for "intellectual disability." Those who fit his typology are often referred to as "Kanner autistics" to indicate the severe degree of their impairment.

Researcher Dr. Lorna Wing summarized Kanner's original theory and his addendum to it 13 years later. In his 1943 paper, she reports, Kanner identified the following core features:

- A profound lack of affective contact with other people

- An anxiously obsessive desire for the preservation of sameness in the child's routines and environment

- A fascination for objects, which are handled with skill in fine-motor movements

- Mutism or a kind of language that does not seem intended for interpersonal communication[109]

Kanner also emphasized onset from birth or before 30 months. In the years since he originated the diagnosis, Kanner and subsequent colleagues in the field have modified the diagnostic criteria by selecting two areas as essential:

- A profound lack of affective contact

- Repetitive and ritualistic behavior, which must be of an elaborate kind

If these two features were present, they reasoned, the rest of the typical clinical picture for autism would also be found.

The term "high-functioning," when applied to a child with autism, refers to the child's IQ and degree of ability to use language. However, the child's symptoms of autism may fall into a "spectrum" from mild to severe. Some children with HFA test with a lower IQ and have more severe problems using language to communicate with others. Other children with HFA may test "average" to "superior" on IQ tests. Though their speech may seem odd and abrupt, their communication skills are sufficient for them to get their needs met at home and do well in school. Many people with the HFA neurotype are very successful even though they may lead secluded lives involved in specialized work. Understanding how HFA and AS are similar and different is important for several reasons.

First, having one or the other diagnosis can make a difference in the educational services the child receives. Many children with AS can succeed in a mainstream environment. However, it is less likely that children with autism will be able to be successful in general education classes because they tend to be exclusive visual learners and have more substantial problems with interpersonal communications and social relationships in general.

The cognitive deficits of some children with autism are so impairing that they will be a focus for special education services and other agencies. School districts will generally be successful at understanding and helping these kids. However, helping children with HFA who may score in the "normal" to "superior" range on IQ tests is more problematic.

Miya, one of my clients, a 16-year-old girl, comes to mind as a good example of this issue. She had been brought to me by her parents with a diagnosis of "Severe ADD (inattentive type) and AS, with severe anxiety, sensory integration problems, and obsessions." Her diagnosticians had decided on the AS and ADD diagnoses because of her extreme inattention, her lack of response to requests by others to communicate with her, and her obsessive needs for safety and predictability. She was receiving home-based tutoring and actively resisted going to school.

While Miya's history could suggest the presence of ADD and AS, there were subtle differences. For example, though she looked directly at me, she seemed to be "wide eyed" in the sense that she was simply looking at everything in front of her, and I was just one of the objects in view. She was extremely inattentive, seeming lost in her own thoughts. Her behavior was not that unusual for someone with OCD, but there was one dramatic thing Miya did that got my attention. Coming into the waiting room in my office to get her, I saw her lying on the floor, face down, with her head under one of the chairs. Her mother sat calmly beside her as if this happened all the time.

I asked Miya if the head-under-the-chair behavior was a protection from sensory overwhelm and she confirmed that hunch. My interview with her also revealed the presence of a powerful social phobia and powerful sensory preferences – by her own design, her room was stark, painted blue, with only a few pieces of furniture present. If anything was disturbed, she became highly anxious.

I used what I called the "Gorilla test" to get a sense of her place on the autism spectrum. That is, I read several of the introductory pages from Dr. Dawn Prince-Hughes' excellent autobiography (she is autistic), *Songs of the Gorilla Nation,*[110] in which she describes her sensory differences, preferences, and aversions. When I finished, I looked up at Miya sitting across from me. She had been silently crying as I read; now she was looking straight at me saying in a matter-of-fact manner, "Yes. That's me. All of it. That's me."

Miya shared our discussion with her parents, who took her to a local autism specialty clinic where she was formally diagnosed with HFA. Her school district Special Education Department was happy to get the information, as many of their attempts to reach her and teach her had been unsuccessful to that point. As it happened, the district was in the process of putting together a program for "visual learners" staffed by people trained to communicate with and teach students with HFA. The program turned out to be a natural fit for Miya, who made a friend there and gradually began coming out of her self-imposed exile at home.

It was Miya's powerfully unfocused communication style, her sense of being lost in her own world, and her behavioral oddities (as suggested in her behavior in the waiting room), that (in my clinical opinion) differentiated her from children with AS. Unlike adolescents with AS who get stuck on one subject or nit-pick a topic to death in a monotonic drawl, or constant whining, Miya said nothing and did not seem to hear much of what I said until I started bridging to her with *Gorilla.* A person with her perceptual style, challenges, and gifts needs a different educational approach than does a person with AS (who may seek so much attention from others that they begin discouraging contact). To be successful, Miya would have to be taught using the kinds of strategies suggested by Dr. Temple Grandin, which are described later in this chapter.

Second, governmental entitlements in terms of education and other services are different for the two diagnoses. AS is not generally considered to be a developmental disability, while autism is. Therefore, those who are diagnosed with autism usually qualify for services. As a child with AS grows through his teens into adulthood, he may not receive the vocational training services he needs because his impairment is not considered severe enough to warrant such services. And the parents sometimes have to fight with the school district to get their child an IEP.

By comparison, children who are more profoundly affected by autism may resist going to school, or, once there, are very difficult to reach and teach. Because they are the targets of bullies and vulnerable to them, they often develop anxiety reactions just at the mention of school. For many children with HFA, it is easier to justify the need for an IEP, as school personnel are more likely to have noticed areas of concern.

Third, HFA and AS children often require different parenting strategies and different approaches in psychotherapy. The child with HFA is less able to escape from the confines of his inner world to communicate effectively with neurotypicals. On the other hand, the child with AS, while he may have poor communication skills, is much less impaired in the ability to make contact with others, to engage in problem solving with them, and to organize his life. Further, a child with AS may be better able to benefit from insight-oriented psychotherapy, whereas the child with HFA may relate to the process as one would who is stranded in a strange country in which everyone else is speaking an unknown language.

A good place to start in getting clearer on the differences between the personalities and challenges of children with these two diagnoses is to look at how the DSM-IV defines autism and Asperger's Disorder.

## How the DSM-IV Differentiates Autism from Asperger Syndrome

We have said that the diagnostic manual labels autism as one of a class of disorders grouped as PDD, which also includes Asperger's Disorder. The DSM-IV description makes clear that autism and AS share two main symptom clusters: "Qualitative impairment in social interaction" and presence of "Restrictive, repetitive, and stereotyped patterns of behavior." But it says that children with autism, unlike those with AS, will show impairments in the development of language and ability to *communicate* with others. Further, the DSM-IV holds that children with autism must have a delay in one or more of the following areas: (a) social communication, (b) language development, and (c) symbolic or imaginal play. This is not specified in the diagnostic criteria for AS.

Nevertheless, the DSM-IV does not provide a clear distinction between autism and AS. It says, in effect, AS and autism are similar except for the fact that children with autism have problems using language, symbolic play (a form of communication), and communicating verbally with others. It does not indicate whether these difficulties will be present in AS, implying, by omission, that they will not. Thus, it does not give us the specificity necessary to clearly identify a child as fitting one diagnosis or another.

Many professionals are able to describe with clarity the behaviors and cognitive processes of people with autism, but they typically do not address the difference between HFA and AS. It is as if everyone is saying, "Well, the DSM-IV says they're different but really they are not. AS is just another term for very high-functioning autism. We all know that, whatever the DSM-IV says." In fact, that ambiguity has been there from the beginning when the diagnosis was described by Dr. Lorna Wing, who stated:

> In the light of this finding, is there any justification for identifying Asperger Syndrome as a separate entity? Until the aetiologies of such conditions are known, the term is helpful when explaining the problems of children and adults who have autistic features, but who talk grammatically and who are not socially aloof.[111]

I interpret Dr. Wing to say that she is willing to put forth the diagnosis of AS because there is a pattern of behavior in evidence that is probably a part of autism but that is being discounted because children with this pattern are not as "obviously impaired." That is, they do not match up to the old idea that children with autism all sit in the corner, mute, playing with dust balls. They need help, but their symptoms are not dramatic enough to get them the help, so we have to assign them a separate diagnosis.

We need to look at the issue with fresh eyes to understand the striking dissimilarities between the two conditions. My clinical experience has taught me that however similar these conditions look, they are very different, and it is important to know this difference if we are going to help children who occupy each neurotype.

Please note that the following observations of differences between HFA and AS are my theories of what these children are experiencing. I provide citations to back up some of the comments I make – what has been demonstrated in research studies – but the construction, the theory, is all my own.

## "Fixed-Figure" vs. "Full-Field" Perceptual Style

In Chapter One, I discussed the idea from Gestalt psychology and developmental psychology that learning involves picking out things as "figure," separate objects of focus from their "background" or "field," focusing on the figural object, learning from it, and then letting it fade into the ground to move on to a new figure. Take, for example, two children who meet for the second time at school. The first time was on a field trip that took place several weeks earlier. If the rhythm of figure-ground is working correctly, one child will first pick the other out from the "field" of several hundred other kids on the playground (making him an initial "figure" in his mind). He will mentally sort the other child out of the "field" of all the other kids he remembers from the outing in which they met, making a "remembered figure" of him. Now he will sort out his feelings and perceptions of this particular person and categorize him as "potential friend" or "forget it." If "potential friend" is chosen, he will talk to the other child and their interaction in the moment will become a new figure, which will later fade into the field of his consciousness of experiences for the day.

**AS perspective.** If a child occupies the AS perceptual style, this meeting will go as follows. First, the child may not open conversation with the other because he or she does not share the perceiver's special interest; that is, is not interested in the mythology of dragons or cell phones, medical equipment, or whatever is "figural" for the child. Alternatively, the child with AS may try to make contact around his special interest. The child with AS is able to make a mental "figure" out of the other child and perhaps note where he met him: "That is a fifth-grader that I remember from the field trip." But if the other child is not interested in the special interest of the child with AS, the interaction will probably stop right there because the child with AS is unable to sort out from his memory of conversations with people a memory of how he started a conversation with a stranger that did not involve his special interest.

If the interaction is forced by an adult, the child with AS may be able to ask a few rehearsed questions but will not be able to carry the conversation because he does not possess a repertoire of suitable comments to make. Building a repertoire requires that at some time in the past, he experienced rewarding social interactions. Because of his tendency to be fixated on his special interest and inability to generalize to the Big Picture, he does not have this repertoire – he does not have a full fund of "figural" social memories to access.

**HFA perspective.** Unlike the child with AS, the child with HFA demonstrates use of a "full-field" perceptual style. In the example we are using here, he will go out onto the playground and see all of the children at once. One Big Picture filled with moving, screaming, running, new smells, conflicts, joy, and bright light. He will not be able to pick out or remember any one particular child. If an adult tries to force a social encounter, the child with HFA may devolve into hysteria or uncontrollable giddiness or may use some perseverant behavior such as holding his ears, rocking, or screaming to calm himself. It is all just too much.

The HFA child sees only the forest (at least at first) and cannot see the individual trees. The AS child sees only One Special Tree (at first) and needs a lot of help generalizing to take in the fact that his tree exists as part of a forest.[111]

Olga Bogdashina, a researcher in the field of autism, writes this about the inability of the child with autism to distinguish between foreground and background:[112]

> There is much evidence that one of the problems many autistic people experience is their inability to distinguish between foreground and background stimuli (inability to filter foreground and background information). They are often unable to discriminate relevant and irrelevant stimuli. What is background to others may be equally foreground to them; they perceive everything without filtration or selection.

Dr. Bogdashina goes on to say:

> Their difficulty to filter background and foreground information caused by Gestalt perception leads to rigidity of thinking and lack of generalization. They can perform in the exactly same situation with the exactly same prompts but fail to apply the skill if anything in the environment, routine, prompt, etc., has been even slightly changed. For example, the child can perform the task if he is being touched on the shoulder and fails if he has not been given the prompt. Or a familiar room may seem different and threatening if the furniture has been slightly rearranged, etc.

### *"Right-Brain" Capability at the Expense of "Left-Brain" Talent*
In Chapter One, I discussed the research that suggests that some children show evidence of a pattern of brain growth in which at some point, between the age of 1 and 3, they become specialized to either the left- or right-brain hemisphere.[113]

I also talked about how the child later diagnosed with AS shows strong left-brain abilities (such as numerical reasoning) and loses right-brain abilities such as the ability to effectively multi-task or form abstract, creative, conclusions from divergent data to Big Picture things.

I hypothesize that as children with HFA go through this process, their brains lose a lot of the left-brain ability to use internal speech and language to break things into parts and sequences. At the same time, these children develop compensatory strengths in terms of right-brain visual thinking abilities. When they become specialized to the right side, children with HFA lose the ability to think in words and many of the other abilities of the left frontal brain, to include the ability to:

- Deal with one sensory input at a time

- Process information in a linear and sequential format

- Accurately track the passage of time (the clock is a device that uses language to communicate its meaning)

- Use language to express inner states, feelings, and beliefs

- Think logically and analytically using language to represent information

At the same time, they gain significant advantage in the following areas:

- Visualizing objects in their minds from many different angles with great accuracy

- Presence of phenomenal visual-feeling memories (we have noted Dr. Dawn Prince-Hughes' contention that she remembers her own birth)

- Ability to remember and mimic things that they have seen

- Recognizing by "a different feel" places, faces, objects, and music

## Four Marked Behavioral Differences Between Children with HFA and Children with AS

The tendency of the child with HFA to take in the world as "full field" and the tendency of the child with AS to take in the world as "fixed figure" has a profound impact on the child's development and the specific challenges that he will experience.

1.  **Infants and young children with HFA and AS behave very differently as they develop.**
    Although it is impossible to identify with certainty the difference between a child with autism (and HFA) from one with AS at an early age, the following checklist summarizes features that have been included in a variety of sources as characterizing each condition.[114]

    A caveat is in order when reading the checklist. The characteristics listed are typical of the development of children with autism but may not be seen in *all* children who fit the autistic or HFA subtypes. For example, some children will not show such dramatic evidence of the detached and uncommunicative perceptual style described. There will be peculiarities in the child's communication process, but there will not be the extreme loss of contact noted. Thus, we could say that applying these developmental criteria may yield a "false negative" – the child may not show these features but may later be diagnosed as autistic. But there is much less likelihood of a "false positive": If these features are present, there is a very high probability that the child has autism.

**Developmental Differences Between Children with HFA and Children with AS, Birth to 14 Months**

| Feature | Feature Present in Autism (and HFA) | Feature Present in Asperger Syndrome |
|---|---|---|
| **Does he follow a finger point with adult instruction "look there"?** | No. He cannot sort out the figures involved – the image of "finger," the words "look there." | Does follow finger-point. Has no problem sorting out the complex details of the situation and following the adult's instruction. |
| **Does he make eye contact with parents and others?** | No. Not only does he not sort out others' eyes as figure, his brain does not ascribe meaning to others' faces apart from background. | Does make eye contact in non-threatening situations. May avoid eye contact if overstressed. |
| **Does he respond to peek-a-boo games?** | No. Everything is seen "full field" and right now, or else it does not exist. There is no "figural memory" of the game from the past. | Yes, but may resist out of disinterest; he does not derive a lot of personal satisfaction from this contact. The child can be socially reciprocal if he has to; however, he often does not initiate social interactions. |

*Note.* These characteristics tend to be present depending on whether a child's diagnosis is "mild," "moderate," or "severe."

## Developmental Differences Between Children with HFA and Children with AS (continued)

| Feature | Feature Present in Autism (and HFA) | Feature Present in Asperger Syndrome |
|---|---|---|
| **Is he speaking in complete sentences by 24 months?** | No and yes. Some HFA children do not acquire language until a year or two past when this milestone is normally met (by age 2). There is a lag in brain development. | Usually. Children with AS are very often precocious verbalizers with huge vocabularies they may only partially understand. |
| **Is his speech odd or unusual sounding?** | Yes. Some may show presence of echolalia, which is the term used to denote repetition of what is heard such as repetition of a teacher's directives or repetition of anything said to him or heard (e.g., favorite movies), repetition of particular words such as "fire truck," "light bulb." | Yes. Will show odd speech prosody; they have unusual pronunciation or vocabulary use but their speech development is usually normal in other ways. They often appear to be delivering little lectures when speaking about many subjects. |
| **Does he like physical contact and rough housing?** | No. This feature is noted on research-based checklists for autism, not in the diagnosis. Only strong, firm touch is felt as "safe." | Sometimes. May enjoy this contact with certain people around whom he feels very safe. |
| **Does he use his index finger to point in order to draw attention to something or ask a question?** | Rarely. This is a gesture used to pick some object of interest out of background or field. The child does share a "joint attention" with his adult caregiver; he may observe the caregiver but does not share an exchange of meaning with her that would naturally lead him to look in the direction of the finger point. | Yes. There is no problem choosing a figure, especially if it is of special interest to the child. |

**Developmental Differences Between Children with HFA and Children with AS (continued)**

| Feature | Feature Present in Autism (and HFA) | Feature Present in Asperger Syndrome |
|---------|-------------------------------------|--------------------------------------|
| **Does he respond to caregiver strategies involving reward and punishment?** | Rarely. Will withdraw, become passive; shows no interest in making authority figures happy with his behavior. To respond to punitive strategy involves the ability to think in words, "I did this yesterday and I was punished. Therefore, I will not do this today." | Yes. Will respond if he sees reward in the situation. Will be loudly oppositional to punishment strategies out of anxiety. (See Chapter Five on ODD for description of the relationship of high anxiety to oppositionality.) |
| **Does he engage in pretend play using toys, such as "having a tea party"?** | No. Does not use symbolic play as communication. This requires recognition of play themes, which requires well-developed mental language ability. | Sometimes. Pretend play may involve a special interest but is rarely symbolic or whimsical. He is very self-centered, precise, and controlling. |
| **Does he head-bang, moan, scream, or use other perseverant behaviors?** | Often. May scream and hold hands over ears. This provides a sense of "self-as-origin" that may be profoundly lacking in a child who does not remember any physical experience. | This feature is also seen in AS but is typically less severe and occurs as a response to frustration more than an attempt to gain a sense of oneself as originator of one's own behavior. |
| **Does he fixate on shiny objects?** | Often. Will seem "lost in pleasant hyperfocus" on these items. HFA children are visual and very soothed by simple visual beauty. | Rarely. However, even very young children with AS may have a special interest. Children with HFA and AS both have an interest in the details of things, but AS children tend to do so because these details are related to a special interest. |

## Developmental Differences Between Children with HFA and Children with AS (continued)

| Feature | Feature Present in Autism (and HFA) | Feature Present in Asperger Syndrome |
|---|---|---|
| Is he oversensitive to textures, smells, sounds, light levels, and crowding? | Very common. May dramatically and suddenly withdraw if overstimulated. This is a result of flooding from full-field perception that is particularly distressing to younger and lower-functioning people with HFA. | In my observation, children with AS are oversensitive to touch, crowding, and sounds made by others. They are less troubled by the other stimuli listed. |
| When did he start acting as if he was "in a world of his own"? | Often normal development proceeded to a "sudden stop" point and then language and communication became problematic. | AS patterns of poor social relationships, self-centeredness, high anxiety, and stereotypical interests and mannerisms were evident from the beginning of his life. No abrupt onset. |
| Does he have a strong resistance to change in routine? | Yes. His reaction may be meltdown or extremely high anxiety. If one aspect of the field changes, the whole internal representation of the field collapses. | Yes. Reaction typically similar but less severe than for children with HFA. This one is also in the diagnosis for AS. |
| Does he take an interest in other children? | Yes, for higher-functioning children. However, HFA-related communication difficulties may make social contact so painful that he withdraws and does not seem interested. | Yes. However, may not know how to express his interest. Though this feature is listed in the diagnosis for AS, these children are better able to sustain communication with other children than are HFA kids, and generally show more interest in play and having friends (writer's clinical observation). |

**Developmental Differences Between Children with HFA and Children with AS (continued)**

| Feature | Feature Present in Autism (and HFA) | Feature Present in Asperger Syndrome |
|---|---|---|
| **Is he well coordinated physically?** | Children with HFA may demonstrate very good right-left coordination in their movements through early elementary school. They may become wooden and poorly coordinated later on. | In my observation, children with AS are more predictably clumsy – they do not move gracefully, but plod along. They tend to walk toes turned out or turned in with a stoop (plodding through a field). |

2. **Unlike children with AS, children with HFA are primarily visual thinkers.**

   Reading Dr. Temple Grandin's assertion in her book *Thinking in Pictures* that autistics and animals are both exclusive visual thinkers prompted me to conduct informal surveys of the children I work with who have each diagnosis.

   I chose nine children in the age range 8-15 who were diagnosed with AS and six who carried a medical diagnosis of autism. At different times in my meetings with these clients, I asked them to help me solve problems, usually involving open-ended questions in which there were no fixed answers. For one child I might ask, "How would you go about designing that hovercraft you are working on for your science project at school? " Alternatively, I might ask, "What would be one way to approach the current hassle you are having with your friend Billy?"

   As my clients answered the questions, I would note their eye movement patterns to get an idea if they were accessing (looking) up right or up left indicating eye movement typically associated with recall and process of images or pictures (see Chapter Four). If, in answering my questions their eyes moved back and forth on the vertical, or if they looked down to the left or right, I hypothesized that they were recovering and processing word strings, sentences, and auditory material. If their eyes moved up to the left or right, I hypothesized that they were recovering visual images in answer to my question. Eye movement in this direction is typically associated with visual recall (up left) or visual planning (up right).[115]

I would then ask them if they saw pictures in their minds or felt they were reading words from a text or writing words as they thought about the problem. Usually they confirmed the impression I already had from their eye movement. Results of this informal study indicated all of the six kids diagnosed with autism and HFA processed all of our transactions visually. Of the nine AS clients, all processed both visually and auditorily, and all showed some problem comprehending information that was only delivered auditorily.

I have always been intrigued by the skills of HFA children who write computer programs. Surely, this is a demonstration of auditory processing. This fact should undermine the idea that children with HFA are exclusive visual processors. True to the writing of Temple Grandin and others, these children approached the job of writing computer code with a visual thinking style. They related that they could "see" lines of computer code as full strings in their minds that displayed themselves as a mental "reader board" or video of the code. Dr. Grandin writes:

> Discussions with other autistic people have revealed visual methods of thinking on tasks that are often considered sequential and nonvisual. A brilliant autistic computer programmer told me that he visualized the entire program tree in his mind and then filled in the program code on each branch. A gifted autistic composer told me that he made "sound pictures." In all these cases, a hazy whole or gestalt is visualized, and the details are added in a non-sequential manner. When I design equipment, I often have a general outline of the system, and then each section of it becomes clear as I add details.[116]

So although it is not in the diagnosis for either autism or AS, I look for evidence that a child is an exclusive visual processor when looking for a diagnosis. Of course, being an exclusive visual thinker does not provide necessary and sufficient evidence that a child fits the HFA neurotype. However, if I see the presence of this predilection, I look closely for other distinguishing features of autism.

There are three ways to detect a child's primary thinking style between thinking in pictures and thinking in words:

- When solving a problem, do his eyes move up right or up left? (These eye movements are associated with visual remembering (up left) and thinking about the future (up right).

- Does he use many visual metaphors ("I see what you mean. I can't really picture that.") or auditory metaphors ("I think I hear you. Let me put that in my own words.")

- Does he report that he always sees pictures when he is solving problems or that thinking is like reading text in the back of his mind?

3. **Unlike the child with AS, the child with HFA may be disabled by overstimulation.**

The inability to separate meaningful figure from background makes the experience of normal levels of stimulation unbearable to a child with HFA. Since she cannot close off her perception to any stimuli, she is subject to hitting the overwhelm point quite quickly in idiosyncratic ways, as exemplified below:

- Although noise levels are no different from usual, she reports pain upon hearing certain noises such as the school buzzer that signals change of classes, the hum of the school's PA system, or the sounds of furniture scraping the floor when the class rearranges itself into workgroups.

- Although the odors in the school cafeteria are no more pronounced than usual, she becomes nauseated at the faint smell of some particular food cooking and refuses to go to the lunchroom for the rest of the year.

- Although she lives in a temperate climate, she experiences ordinary sunlight as painful and must wear polarizing glasses at all times when outside.

- Although the school is not overcrowded with children, she panics when having to walk in a crowd from one classroom to another, goes to the nurse's office and will not come out. She feels like everyone is coming at her at once.

- She may have eating hypersensitivity – experience intense sensations as she chews and swallows certain foods, and swallowing some foods disgusts her. She cannot dissociate from certain feelings, such as the sensation of food going down her throat. Normally people "turn off" this kind of awareness. But taking all sensation in as "full field," she cannot shut off the tendency to make figure out of the feeling of noodles going into her stomach.

- Because she cannot sense the feeling of someone touching her skin as a separate localized event ("I feel someone touching me on my upper arm"), she becomes extremely uncomfortable with any touch at all. Light touch on her arm, for example, may send very unpleasant sensations of tickling all over her arms and back. To compensate for the inability to tolerate touch from others, she may seek very firm pressure in any touch she experiences.

Children with HFA tell me that they are unable to tolerate normal stimulation. They may also experience painful feelings of being emotionally and physically "numb and lifeless" inside as a chronic inner state. They cannot get a sense of stimulus satisfaction from anything. They are caught in a nowhere zone between too much stimulation from the outside and no sense of stimulus satisfaction inside themselves. This painfully contradictory state of sensation deprivation moves some children with HFA to extreme sensory practices. The HFA child may create an environment in his room that most kids would consider suffocating. He puts down the shades, turns up the heat, and turns off the lights. Another child with HFA might enjoy going out late at night when the colors are cool in black and white and there are no people around. Some children go further, giving themselves pinpoint electrical stimulation or engaging in self-cutting or substance use.

Although children with AS may show unusual sensory aversions and cravings, there is a noticeable degree of difference in severity between AS and HFA in this regard. For example, although he may be very uncomfortable in high-stress environments such as a crowded, noisy, smelly, classroom, the child with AS is typically better able to tolerate the stress and stay in the room using his verbal communication skills to make caregivers change the setting. Although high stress may be difficult for him, he is able to have enough of a sense of himself and others at the same time, and therefore is able to communicate his feelings and thoughts to others. As a diagnostician, I pay attention to these differences in degree.

4. **Children with HFA use repetitive self-soothing behaviors to give themselves a sense of existence, of being the source of their own actions. Children with AS use repetitive behaviors to reduce stress.** Both children with HFA and children with AS show repetitive, ritualistic types of behavior (apart from compulsions associated with OCD). Children with HFA exhibit such behaviors as groaning, head banging, jumping repetitively, spinning, staring into space, or staring at shiny objects. Though these full-body movements are not as typical among children with AS, these kids will head-bang or slap themselves frequently. It is important to understand the function that these behaviors have for a child when trying to differentiate AS from HFA.

My clinical observation is that children with HFA demonstrate perseverant self-soothing behaviors to give themselves a sense of origin in their lives. I came upon this reason in the excellent Appendix to Donna Williams' book *Nobody Nowhere,* in which she makes clear that all these behaviors remind a child who has no autobiography that he is a body, a unique person separate from the field in which he exists.

Subvocally, the child says to himself as he jumps, "This is me jumping and this is me experiencing the predictability of the shock that rises through my body from my feet when I hit the floor." Or repetitively dropping an object, the preschool HFA child says to himself, "This is me dropping this ball and picking it up.[117]

Because the child does not think in words, he cannot hold a memory of physical experience; he cannot experience a sense of personal identity. Repetitive and ritualistic behaviors give him the otherwise missing sense of the flow of events, of time, of place, and of his own participation as an anonymous human being in the life of the world.

Perseverant behaviors may also be very specific reactions to specific sensory threats that cause the child to experience high anxiety. Here again we see sensory overload caused by his full-field perceptual style – he cannot sort it all out and deal with it one stimulus at a time.

- He may hold his hands over his ears to screen out a noise, ordinary to everyone else, that is causing him intolerable pain.

- He may choke himself in class to dull himself to the anxiety he feels from being forced to interact emotionally with other children in the classroom.

- He may pull his coat over his head and face and refuse to remove it to deal with the extreme anxiety he experiences from the noise, light, crowding, and smells at school.

In my observation, children with AS use repetitive and ritualistic behavior to relieve stress, not to give themselves a sense of "self-as-origin" as seen in HFA. A child with AS may hit herself in the head or bang her head on the desk, but this is typically a response to some particular frustration as if to say "Why can't you just get this through your stupid head?" The perseverant behavior serves to sidetrack the anxiety the child feels for a few moments and absolve her of guilt. These are important positive outcomes for the child.

Thus, a behavior that serves to give the child with AS relief from stress and anxiety may serve to give the child with HFA a sense of identity. This is an important distinction. Unlike the child with HFA, the child with AS is able to use mental language (e.g., self-talk) to remember himself as a person, to remember a mythic autobiography that answers the questions: "Who am I? Who are all these others? and What are we doing together?"

---

### Four Differences Between Children with HFA and Children with AS

1. There are striking differences in the way in which infants and young children with HFA and AS behave as they develop.

2. Unlike children with AS, children with autism are primarily visual thinkers.

3. Unlike the child with AS, the child with HFA may be disabled by overstimulation.

4. Children with HFA use repetitive self-soothing behaviors to give themselves a sense of existence, of being the source of their own actions. Children with AS use repetitive behaviors to reduce personal stress and anxiety.

---

## Four Success Strategies for Parenting Children with AS or HFA

Generally speaking, any parenting or educational strategy that helps an AS child be more successful also helps the child with HFA.

The child with AS is challenged by greatly impaired social ability, a lack of empathy, and difficulty focusing on anything other than a special interest, but he does not suffer many of the cognitive challenges of the child with HFA. Some children with AS may be taught in a general education classroom. Some will need more one-to-one assistance. Most will need intense social skills mentoring at school. With these accommodations, most children with AS as a stand-alone condition are able to learn in mainstream or "advanced placement" classrooms.

It is generally more difficult for children with HFA to keep up in a mainstream environment. The HFA child's visual and full-field perceptual style may cause her to experience severe communication problems and isolate her. The extreme stress of being in a crowded, noisy environment will exert pressure on the child to close down and run away. More important, the HFA child often simply does not understand what is required of her. She will not understand the meaning of some words, classroom lectures, and how to take tests. Schools are environments created by and for people who think in words. This may leave the child with HFA feeling as if she is stranded on an unfamiliar planet.

Once you have a clearer idea of the neurotype of the child, you are in a position to help her get the specialized help that she needs. The basic challenge for the child with HFA is to stay in contact with the world of neurotypicals and persevere in pursuit of her goals in the face of an overwhelming urge to flee and withdraw into her internal world. The basic challenge for the child with AS is to get her needs met in the world of neurotypicals, to fit in well enough so that her "oddness" becomes a selling point.

1. **Challenge the self-centeredness of children with HFA and AS by building a logical and visual sense of community responsibility.** Children diagnosed with AS and with HFA need to remain engaged in the world for their own good. As Dr. Daniel Siegel points out, positive social interaction is an essential requirement for the development of the human nervous system.[118]

    Caregivers prepare a child with HFA and AS for the future by helping him develop ways to respond to demands from "the world."

    • *Pre-school-aged children with HFA and AS* benefit from regular participation in games involving turn taking. This helps them get the idea that they are members of a group and if everyone in the group is to get a chance at the game, everyone must pause and watch from time to time.

    • Younger children with HFA should be required to participate in family rituals such as household cleanup, dinner, and outings. Time should be taken to teach them how to do these things. It will take a lot more time to do so, but the child with HFA can learn to make his own bed and do his own laundry. It is important to post visual images that remind him of what is required and to drill, drill, and drill again, until he masters the task.

    • If a child needs to reduce stress and assert identity with self-stimulating behaviors (provided these are safe), this should happen at a regularly scheduled time every day.

- *Elementary school-age children with HFA* may benefit from having the concept of community and interdependence explained to them in very concrete terms. Some activities that can be used to visually and concretely depict the concept of community follow.

  - Provide an ant farm to illustrate how the ants work together on a common purpose to improve and upgrade their underground dwelling.

  - Draw a large circle on the floor with masking tape. Inside the circle set up stations that will be occupied by children who each have a part in putting together some project that would not be complete without everyone's participation.

  - The concept of community may also be explained by reference to hierarchies in animal communities or by reference to mythical figures that may have captured the child's imagination, such as characters in the Harry Potter books. To make these concepts concrete and understandable to children with HFA, have them build dioramas containing figures that represent characters in the hierarchy and explain how these characters interact.

- *For older children,* take field trips to the local zoo and assign students the task of observing groups of animal species to report to the class later evidence observed of social interaction among peers, protective behavior, followership, and leadership.

- Teach elementary- and high-school-age children the rudiments of team sports by running them through each position played on a sports team without other players present. HFA children can play team sports, but they must first learn everything there is to know about a position in the game. For example, to teach an HFA adolescent how to play basketball, a coach, parent, special education mentor may spend time after school each day for weeks teaching the child how to play the free throw line, or guard, or how to run and throw the ball from under the hoop. Everything takes more time. There is nothing wrong with repetition as a learning strategy. It is an essential ingredient of progress for children challenged by both HFA and AS.

Once the basics of connection with the community, of kindness, and interdependence are taught to a child with HFA and AS, he may be ready to gain a more complex understanding of community and how he fits in. Caregivers must be very patient and persistent when instructing the HFA child in this abstract concept. They must keep in mind that he does not think in words, cannot form abstractions based on words, and has only the most primitive idea of how people relate together.

To begin, talk with the child while drawing a picture of your idea of how people interact in a *community*. Show what they *get* and *give* to each other. Illustrate the idea of "community responsibility," which means, "You give certain things to the community and you get certain things from the community." Use the child's family or his classroom as examples of how people are interdependent in communities – they have to depend on each other for certain things.

You may want to get more personal with your explanation by drawing cartoon[119] panels using stick figures that illustrate his interaction with the community in some way. For example, you might show him giving certain things to his family community – his energy, his help with daily chores, his wisdom, his tutoring of his little brother. In return, he gets certain things, including the company of others in his family who love him, encouragement, and his needs for daily living are met.

At school, you might draw him sitting around a table working on a project with a couple of his friends. You might illustrate how he provides the "facts" and "useful data" for solving the problem and how one of his neurotypical friends provides the humor that makes the work easier. Describe the idea that a community is a gathering of people who commune together, who interact toward achieving a certain purpose, and that like any mechanical or physical system (illustrate by reference to science), in a community, you take things out and put things in as everyone works toward a desired outcome.

Then give him a few examples such as the behavior of cars at a four-way stop (people have learned rules of politeness to keep things moving). Or describe how we pay taxes to the government and get things back like law enforcement and health services. As you go through these examples, make sure to illustrate any spoken concepts with drawings and pictures.

In my clinical experience, children with HFA have more difficulty understanding the idea of community than children with AS. Living "in a world of his own," feeling very much like the lone resident of a planet, the HFA child may not be able to picture in his mind how people should relate to each other socially. He will not have a model of optimum functioning of people in groups. He needs help in picturing himself as a member of a group and defining the best way to relate to the group

*Children and adolescents with AS and HFA take a lot out of the community. They have a tendency to melt down when stressed. Children with AS may use loud and insulting, kinglike, language when something they want to do is interrupted. These demonstrations deprive the family community of peace of mind. They have taken something out and, in keeping with the give-and-take model of community, must do something to restore balance in the family. Restitution (giving back) has to take place so that reconciliation (bringing everyone together again) may occur.*

*Go over this concept many times: If one takes something out of the community, there must be a giveback. This must occur before things are back the way they "should be."*

Get other communities into the child's life. Participation with other children in activities of mutual interest is greatly stabilizing to children with HFA and AS. Examples of potential communities include:

- Immediate and extended family
- Classmates and the professional staff at school
- Employees of the local grocery store where he works
- The local Boy Scout troop
- Personal and online friends and gaming opponents
- Church or spiritual community, to include its teachers

In the Introduction, I suggested that children with AS and HFA carry a very specific genius, a guiding spirit, that has gifts for the world. The presence of teachers other than parents or primary caregivers is required if a child is to live in genius in the world. Parents cannot do it all because they are parents – and to some extent must share their child's issues. They provide the initial field for his development. Their love, devotion, firmness, and honesty give him ground to stand on. However, the child needs other teachers to get him through crisis points that may be invisible to his parents.

Once an infraction is stated in terms of the family-as-community model, it becomes easier to establish a consequence for any behavior. If you take something out of the community, you must give something in kind back to it. This is not punishment. It is instruction in the reality of "this follows that." It is the parents' willingness to walk the talk – they put effort and care into teaching children who isolate easily from others that they are answerable to their community for their actions.

Here are several examples of the use of the restitution and reconciliation approach:

*Situation:* The child damages some part of the family community (such as punching a hole in the wall).
*Solution:* The child repairs the damage. He may need help such as a caregiver paying for most of the repair material; however, it is important that his part comes out of his allowance.

*Situation:* The child takes the peacefulness from the community by tormenting his sibling.
*Solution:* The child does not receive benefit from others (such as his mom chauffeuring him around) for a period of time.

Children diagnosed with HFA and AS can be quite pragmatic when it comes to getting their way with their parents. For example, they are typically willing to comply with a requirement if a *quid pro quo* is included that is acceptable. Many carry features of OCD and therefore obey the OC command introject to "even things up." Everything is done in twos. Everything must be perfectly balanced. Jump here twice – jump there twice. Therefore, the idea of family community governed by the rule of this-for-that naturally fits their OC personality type.

## 2. Work with the child to co-create a positive Great Story.

To help the HFA or AS child form a positive story for her life, make time every day to listen to her and weave in archetypal themes that are seen in the lives of people with HFA or AS.

The important thing is to listen to a child's story, note the formative events in her life, and wait for the story line to begin to form. In *Genius! Nurturing the Spirit of the Wild, Odd, and Oppositional Child*,[120] I describe how Dr. Temple Grandin went about building a personal autobiography of her success in life. Unable to hold an auditory, word-based memory, she devised a uniquely visual way of marking milestones in her life. She visualized herself going through certain *doors* at certain times. She writes:

> The big challenge for me was making the transition from high school to college. People with autism have tremendous difficulty with change. In order to deal with a major change such as leaving high school, I needed a way to rehearse it, acting out each phase in my life by walking through an actual door, window, or gate. When I was graduating from high school, I would go and sit on the roof of my dormitory and look up at the stars and think about how I would cope with leaving. It was there I discovered a little door that led to a bigger roof (being built) while my dormitory was being remodeled ...When I was in college, I found another door to symbolize getting ready for graduation. I had to actually practice going through this door many times. When I finally graduated from Franklin Pierce College, I walked through a third, very important, door on the library roof.

About her graduation from college, Grandin notes:

> I went through the little door tonight and placed the plaque on the top of the library roof. I was not as nervous this time. I had been much more nervous in the past. Now I had

already made it and the little door and the mountain had already been climbed. *The conquering of this mountain is only the beginning for the next mountain.*[121]

In this last sentence, you see how Grandin created her own Great Story using her powerful visual intelligence to overcome the difficulty that she experienced holding a thought-based memory of her life. Employing this method, she was able to link completion of one stage in her development with the beginning of the next stage. She illustrates how visual autobiography can carry the same power as an auditory autobiography.

Build on Dr. Grandin's wisdom with your HFA child by working with him to imagine visual markers for progress in his life and to get in touch with these markers in a very real sense:

- To help the child recognize his talents, take pictures of him enjoying his favorite things, playing his video games, doing science, or arranging his room with all his animals lined up. Make him a personal photo album with narrative. If you use a digital camera, you can easily put these images onto a CD-ROM, possibly as video that shows him enjoying his various gifts from making music and doing science, to arranging his room "just so."

- Bring to mind five successful events and describe them to him in very visual terms as both of you draw them on clipboards in front of you, or simply describe each event and ask him how it felt to be at that time and place in his life.

- Apply Grandin's method to helping the child envision the future to decrease his resistance to change. If he is to attend a new school, arrange with his building principal to walk him through his daily journey from his room to other places in the school several times over a week or two and make note of specific visual things to look for in the building along the way. Consider Grandin's use of important symbolic physical doorways to help him move from elementary school to middle school to high school and beyond.

3. **Teach a system of visual organization to help the child with HFA and AS understand others' emotional language and motivations.**

Some, not all, children with AS have a difficult time decoding others' emotional language. Typically, there is a feeling of "bemusement" in their observations of others' emotional states – they do not quite get where other people are coming from emotionally, but they are generally able to repair interpersonal communication and maintain the continuity of contact.

Brain scan research conducted by Dr. Simon Baron-Cohen and his colleagues suggests that the brains of people diagnosed with autism and AS are less efficient when it comes to recognizing faces and reading facial expressions of others. (This research did not differentiate autism from AS. It included them together, as is the practice with a lot of research in this area.)[122]

Baron-Cohen detected that the amygdala, the brain's emotional center, did not activate when his subjects viewed expressions of emotion in another's eyes whereas in neurotypical subjects, it did activate.

Because HFA children think in pictures, they often have a difficult time decoding the enormous percentage of communication that is conveyed by changing tone of voice, crying, yelling, and the nonverbal behavior that accompanies these states. Neurotypicals use language to describe their emotional states. Language is used to teach children what certain facial expressions mean. If a child does not have the "onboard translator," the ability to think in words, he is not able to develop a knowledge base for interpreting feelings.

The good news is that children with HFA can learn how to read facial expressions and describe basic emotional states. Unlike children with AS, kids with HFA must learn more than just the mechanics of "acting normally" in a social situation. They have to learn discrete, specific, concrete ways to decode and respond to human emotional communication.

To help AS and HFA children decode others' emotional meanings, teach them how to visually sort pictures of nonverbal behaviors and assign them to "mind files" that describe certain emotional states. Use their excellent ability to take in the detail of an object of interest by first asking them to study photographs of people in their family. Have them use these photographs to describe various ways that these others communicate nonverbally. Then work with them to identify an emotion that is paired with a certain behavior. "When my mom's mouth turns down and her eyes squint, she is either angry or very sad and about to cry."

Attempt to have them identify this feeling in themselves. "When my grandma died, I felt sad." Once the child has identified a set of emotional states for a certain person, ask her to visualize some type of file container in her mind and assign a name to the container such as "mom when sad." Then ask her to "drag and drop" the nonverbal behaviors associated with Mom being sad into that file. When the child sees these behaviors again, she can scan the files in her mind to locate the one containing the appropriate nonverbal behavior. Understanding what the other is experiencing, the child is able to deliver an appropriate response such as a look of "kindness and concern" (a gesture taught using a mirror).

4. **Deal with adolescent issues around sex in a very concrete fashion.**
Boys and girls with AS and HFA need to have the facts of life explained in very clear, understandable terms, with no assumptions being made about their level of sophistication. Some children with AS and HFA have low sexual desire – they are less concerned about it or are neutral about the topic. These adolescents tend to be woefully uninformed and very inexperienced. In addition, because of their lack of social pragmatics, they are at risk of being exploited by unscrupulous neurotypicals. That is, the isolation and loneliness that they experience may make them less careful about people who profess they are "friends."

Younger children also need guidance to protect themselves from being inappropriately touched by older kids as well as adults. The finer nuances of safe and unsafe touch are explained in the children's book *A Very Touching Book*.[123] This book may be used with kids as old as 12. As is the case in explaining anything to a child with AS, anticipate his visual processing style by having a clipboard with lots of paper for spontaneous drawing to explain concepts.

In my practice, a small percentage of boys through middle-school age show gender identity peculiarities. For example, they may imitate the effeminate gestures of girls or have dolls and get into combing their hair, but they do not have a sexual orientation to males and are not particularly interested in sex per se. It is the mimicry of the gentler nature of girls and the attention the boys get from this mimicry that move some of them to pursue an interest in "living the life of a female."[124]

## Creating a Successful School Environment for Children with AS or HFA

Educators generally suspect that a child has a learning disability if her academic achievement is below expectations for her ability level as measured on an IQ test.

I have suggested that children with HFA (and some with AS) have a difficult time understanding material presented auditorily. Because so much of course content is delivered in the auditory modality, many kids with HFA (and quite a few with AS) will test as "learning disabled" from the starting gate.

Typically, children with HFA favor the visual-feeling way of thinking and encounter problems when given instruction in another modality, such as by teacher direction. Children with AS also tend to be visual thinkers, but as we have pointed out, they demonstrate a large vocabulary and are able to do well in coursework that requires high auditory intelligence such as in Latin or the sciences.

Many HFA and AS kids balance a disability in one sense with an above-average ability in another. Here are some examples of this kind of selective pattern of talents:

- A child diagnosed with a NLD may have a very difficult time making meaning of others' nonverbal behavior and may have an equally difficult time forming abstractions from what he sees, but he may have a phenomenal memory for details and rote memorization.

- A child diagnosed with AS may not understand figures of speech, such as "Don't go ballistic on me" or "What is your hunch about that problem?" or "Is (some depressing aspect of his life) that getting you down today?". These kids also have a very difficult time reading others' emotional states. But balancing these impairments may be a greatly enhanced memory for what the child reads or sees, what some would term a "photographic" memory.

Children with AS and HFA can function at a very high level given the opportunity to solve problems their way. They may be "learning disabled" in the classroom, but may be excellent learners in other environments. A more appropriate term to describe them would be "specialized learners." They tend to specialize in real-world types of problems and hands-on learning. Many of them disdain "toys," the kinds of manufactured plastic things you buy in a toy store. They want "real tools," to quote the girlhood demand of Barbara McClintock, who went on to become Dr. Barbara McClintock, and win the Nobel Prize for her research in medicine and physiology in 1983. As a girl, Barbara's special interest was corn and everything about corn. Later, it was her research on the genetics of corn that led to her Nobel Prize. Her discoveries paved the way for the Human Genome Project, completed in 2003, which has led to the identification of over 20,000 human genes.[125]

It is impossible to say for sure if Dr. McClintock fit the AS neurotype, but her possession of a decidedly unemotional personality, her distain of small talk, and her special interest suggest similarity to AS.

It is important that the school environment of children with AS and HFA is appropriate for their learning style. According to the IDEA, or Individuals with Disabilities Education Act, every child is entitled to a "free and appropriate education." Here are three strategies for creating educational settings that are appropriate for children with HFA and AS.

1. **Use results from IQ tests to spot cognitive challenges of autism and HFA.**

   Getting appropriate educational services for a child with AS or HFA requires a solid analysis of her educational needs and any learning disabilities. Because most educational assessments include IQ testing, it is helpful to briefly recap a few important facts from our discussion of IQ testing in Chapter Three.

   A child's IQ expresses the ratio between her mental age and chronological age. A 10-year-old with an IQ of 150 is said to be capable of performing at the cognitive level of an average 15-year-old. The *Wechsler III Test of Intelligence*, the instrument most often used in U.S. schools to set up an IEP, measures IQ in two categories: Verbal IQ, which is essentially a measure of a person's proficiency in language and language-based analysis and reasoning; and Performance IQ, which assesses a person's strength in thinking visually and problem solving. IQ is measured in each area with a set of subtests. The tests may be summarized as follows:

*Verbal Subtests*
- Information: factual knowledge, long-term memory, recall
- Similarities: abstract reasoning, verbal categories and concepts
- Arithmetic: attention and concentration, numerical reasoning
- Vocabulary: language development, word knowledge, verbal fluency
- Comprehension: social and practical judgment, common sense
- Digit Span: short-term auditory memory, concentration

*Performance Subtests*
- Picture Completion: alertness to detail, visual discrimination
- Coding: visual-motor coordination, speed, and concentration
- Picture Arrangement: planning logical thinking, social knowledge
- Block Design: spatial analysis, abstract visual problem solving
- Object Assembly: visual analysis and construction of objects
- Symbol Search: visual-motor quickness, concentration, persistence, scanning
- Mazes: fine-motor coordination, planning, following directions

Research indicates that there is no standard cognitive profile as measured on IQ tests that differentiates AS from HFA, and most research studies lump the two diagnoses together. This research has provided information about how kids with "autism and high-functioning autism" learn and what gets in the way of their learning (AS is most often simply considered to be a subset of autism). This information is useful for educational planning.[125]

This research suggests:

- Children with HFA are visual learners. They typically do better on Performance IQ than children with AS because this part of the test measures visual problem-solving ability.

- Children with HFA do not show deficits in simple memory, simple language, and visual-spatial capability.[126]

- Problems with language comprehension and social reasoning are more marked with the HFA group than with neurotypicals – they have lower scores on the "comprehension" subtest.[127]

- Unlike children with ADD, children with HFA do not encounter significant problems with short-term memory as measured by the Digit Span subtest in the Verbal IQ, but they do show problems remembering lists and other written/auditory information.[128]

- Children with HFA typically show higher scores on problems involving visual reasoning. They will do well on the Block Design subtest in the Performance category.[129]

- Younger children diagnosed with HFA have lower Verbal IQ scores but these catch up with performance scores as they grow into adolescence.[130]

- Children diagnosed with HFA have difficulty with writing, both in the mechanical aspect of putting pen to paper and in the organization of what they wrote. There was a marked difficulty in completing any kind of long report or analytical writing assignment.[131]

Children who showed language development characteristic of AS, or who were diagnosed with AS, had generally better Verbal IQ than the neurotypical or "visual HFA" population. Children with AS tend to have higher Verbal than Performance IQ scores. They tell a good story, but getting the job done is something else.

2. **To prevent social isolation and loss of momentum for change, appoint a "guiding hand" to help children with HFA and AS.**
The person occupying the role of GH is a staff member the child trusts who can help with self-organization, task completion, and homework planning, and be a sympathetic ear and coach for issues involving social pragmatics. To restate a central thesis of this book, good relationship with others is a requirement for the development of the neurological system. A caregiver in the role of GH makes sure that AS and HFA children are not lost and isolated at school.
A person in this role may serve as a "team advisor" to a small

group of children who remain together and meet as a team at least once a month for the entire school year. These meetings provide opportunities for children to go over common problems and support each other. Given the difficulty of integrating children with AS and HFA into social groups, it makes sense to load the situation for success by having children diagnosed with AS or HFA meet with more emotionally competent neurotypicals.

The GH should be able to communicate in visual and logical language and have a good understanding of the special psychiatric issues and neurobiological discomforts that HFA and AS children experience every day. The adult will not try to get the child to "share" his feelings. Sharing of feelings is an inappropriate strategy for all autistic children and some kids with AS, and will just cause the child to feel more isolated and more stressed.

## 3. Set up an autism-friendly classroom environment.[132]

Results from IQ testing and other tests used in educational settings help the child's IEP team plan learning activities that meet her particular, idiosyncratic challenges. Every child is different and must be considered as a person with her own hopes, fears, gifts, and challenges apart from her diagnosis. That being said, my clinical experience tells me that there are differences in what each neurotype needs at school and that a careful analysis of the factors above will help educators get a sense of the child's fit into the "autistic" and HFA template or the AS template. There are subtle but important distinctions that must be taken into account.

We have noted how the HFA child's full-field perceptual style causes him to lose his bearings at school and become extremely anxious as a result. Therefore, in the best learning environment for children with HFA:

- All information is presented visually and illustrated pictorially.

- Lecture is kept to an absolute minimum and avoids abstractions.

- The classroom is set up to minimize stress due to over- or understimulation.

- The language of instruction is logical, clear, and descriptive, and avoids abstractions.

- There is a lot of one-to-one contact.

- Verbal instructions do not exceed three steps in a sequence, and each of these is illustrated.

- There are enough computers in the room for all students to use when writing assignments.

- Children are shown or led through movements that illustrate words. To illustrate "up," for example, the teacher climbs up on classroom furniture. To teach a child how to tie his shoes, the teacher paces the child by putting her hands on his and leading him through the process enough times for him to be able to do it himself.

- Attention is paid to the importance of reducing flickering lights and fluorescent light. Laptops are preferred over desktop computer monitors because their screens have less flicker.

- Handouts are done on different-colored paper for different subjects and lettering is large and bold.

## Eight Essential Strategies for Reaching and Teaching Children with HFA and AS

The HFA children I work with teach me that the cognitive challenges they face, the inability to shift focus, and the feeling that they are stuck in a sensorily hostile universe, make their experience of the world quite different from that of children with AS. Though they may share many specific learning issues with children with AS, they are much less capable of taking care of themselves at school – they are much more impaired by the stress that they experience just getting through each day.

Children with AS are also challenged by the academic issues noted above. In addition, many of them experience problems processing what is said to them. This condition, termed a central auditory processing (CAP) disability, is seen in other neurotypes, including HFA and ADD.

Due to their "fixed-figure" perceptual style, many children with AS are assigned to highly structured classrooms. A major problem will be the child's tendency to talk aloud about his special interest. And he may easily get stuck in hyperfocus on things. His penchant for details will get him in trouble.

A change in teachers might not distress a neurotypical child, but it can throw a child with AS into a tailspin, as does a change in the school's daily schedule or any abrupt change in the child's routine. All of these dynamics make life difficult for the AS child who may flee the scene or melt down if things get too stressful.

Any intervention that helps children with autism will also help a child with HFA. In both situations, the underlying teaching philosophy must be sensitivity to the difference in the child's perceptual style and great care to ensure that he understands what is communicated to him.

## 1. Use an autism- and AS-friendly classroom communication style.

- Know what you want to say before you say it.

- Say it clearly, concisely, visually, and in a "matter-of-fact" tone.

- Stop talking if you observe stereotypical behavior such as hand flapping or humming.

- To ensure effective communication and comprehension, be visual, use clipboard drawings, photos, or sign language.

- Know that background stress and noise will prevent communication. He cannot screen out extraneous stimuli.

- Do not always expect a response or "Thank you."[133]

- Paula Kluth, a teacher who works with autistic children, provides four very useful suggestions for effective communication:

  - Do not insist on eye contact.

  - Consider playing with your voice volume or tone. Put on an accent. Whisper. Sing.

  - Experiment with indirect communication: (a) talk your message quietly to his side while he is watching TV, (b) look away or at the floor when you are speaking, and (c) put an object between the two of you and let conversation happen around his interest in the object.

— Help the child understand language: (a) appoint a neurotypical child to help the autistic child understand figures of speech, (b) double-check to make sure that directions are understood, (c) encourage learning about metaphors – ask for "today's metaphor" illustrated with pictures of the metaphor such as a picture of someone "flying off the handle" or "sitting on the fence," and (d) encourage students to keep a personal encyclopedia of puzzling language.[134]

2. **Use a shorthand system to check in with the child on her state of mind and feelings from time to time during the day.**
   Because it is difficult for neurotypical caregivers always to be logical, simple, and visually descriptive in their language, it is often useful to use scales and binary (choice between two alternatives) communication. Using a scale, the teacher simply gives the child a range of 1-7 for a certain characteristic and asks her to indicate her answer by saying a number on the scale. "On a scale of 1-7 where 7 equals 'terrified' and 1 equals 'no problem whatsoever,' what is it like for you to go into the lunchroom at fourth period?" Or, using the binary approach, "Please give me a 'yes' or 'no' answer to the following question: 'I understand why my math teacher gets mad at me?'"

3. **Practice the rule of indirectness to get through to a child with HFA or AS.**
   Children with AS have problems with direct criticism from caregivers because of their difficulty interpreting nonverbal behavior and their tendency to misconstrue the meaning of others, but they can take some direct communication if it is delivered carefully and politely.

   Children with HFA, however, may become highly anxious if confronted. They do not understand verbal instructions or expressions of emotion and become painfully confused if they feel that they are being forced to respond to a situation that is unintelligible to them. To avoid such reactions, develop skill in indirect communication – talking out the window or as if someone else was musing about your situation with you in the room.

   A teacher may observe, for example, that a child withdraws to the back of the room, placing himself with his back to the wall under a desk when other children in the class are milling around in preparation for getting into new work teams. Instead of confronting the child directly about his noncompliance, she goes over, sits next to him on the floor facing outward, and begins describing what she sees from this perspective and how she understands how hard it is for him to stay focused when the whole "field" of the classroom is changing. It is all so confusing. He is receptive to her because she has achieved rapport with his perceptual style and is open to discussing ways that bring him back into the class work after things have settled down and it is perceptually safe for him to do so.

4. **Know the many faces of HFA and AS in children.**
   Teachers who work with children with autism should be able to use the communication strategies noted above as second nature. The best teacher knows that communication is the most important thing and that the teacher's job does not involve trying to get an autistic child to behave as a neurotypical, including making good eye contact and engaging in small talk. The best teacher for this population knows that stress causes oppositionality and comes up with ways to communicate with the child, learn what stresses her, and reduce them.

   The best teacher understands the multiple challenges faced by students with HFA, including extremes of preference for visual, logical, and concretistic thought patterns, high anxiety, and obsessionality. This teacher helps the child overcome the terrors she experiences trying to accommodate her needs given these differences. The teacher does not label her as oppositional defiant or "behaviorally disturbed," but understands barriers to performance and removes these barriers.

   Staff should also be able to deal with the high anxiety, talkativeness, impulsivity, and auditory processing issues of the child with AS. This includes using the child's special interest as the primary vehicle for teaching him and making his competence in that special interest part of his classroom identity: "Quick, someone get Norm. We need help with the network and he's the only one who knows it well enough!" Not only should children with AS and HFA be accorded special status for their gifts, they must be protected by tough-minded control of the school's bullies.

5. **Teach children with HFA by bracketing concept instruction with practical examples.**

   Use the practical "example sandwich" – a strategy I have developed to help kids with HFA take in and use subject matter. That is, before explaining any concept or idea, introduce it with a specific example. Then deliver the concept and illustrate it with another specific example. Then return to the specific, concrete example with a question to the student such as "Is that clear?" The best teachers avoid use of figures of speech and other abstract language when communicating with kids with AS and HFA.

6. **Use "talk-aloud" to demonstrate appropriate social behaviors.**

   Using this instructional method, teachers model appropriate social behaviors and explain them in simple, specific, matter-of-fact language. Teachers "talk aloud" the mental processes they go through when making decisions or interacting with each other. The kids in class are invited to comment on the motivation and the social behavior of teachers, and teachers encourage students to correlate and remember the meaning of specific verbal and nonverbal behaviors.

   For example, to illustrate the importance of giving others privacy, two teachers might talk to each other in front of the class as follows:

   > Al: "John, I walked by your office today and your door was open. I thought of coming in, but then noticed that you had your chair turned away from the door and you were looking out the window. I figured that you were doing that to give yourself freedom from interruption from other people because I had to talk to your back. So I kept going down the hall to my office. What was going on for you?"
   > John: "Al, you had it right. I was trying to solve a problem and did not want to be interrupted. I should have closed my door. I had it open because I have said that I have an 'open door policy,' but that time I needed to be alone with my own thoughts."

   Talking aloud is a good teaching tool because children with AS and HFA cannot mentalize; they cannot make accurate assumptions about others' intent. The method makes clear and concrete how another thinks and solves problems.

7. **Provide concrete and visual ways for students to know exactly what they are expected to do at any particular time and how to determine when a task is completed.**

- Use a visual task scheduler. This is a three-ring-type binder or similar system that gives the child a place to move a card from one place in the binder to another, indicating that a task is completed. (Instructing a student on his morning class schedule: "Eddie, when you complete your reading assignment for the day in the Crafton history book, make sure to move your card to the completed folder. Then go to the next one in the "To do today" folder, which will be your math problems. OK?"

- Provide accurate models of what a school project looks like when complete. Samples of completed-to-requirement written work should be provided. If it is a science project, students should have the opportunity to examine a mock-up of a project that meets your requirements.

- Use different-colored paper for different topic areas.

Teens with HFA and AS have difficulty scheduling their work and need to receive it on a fixed time line with evaluation at identified points in the course. Coursework must be chunked into modules and evaluated before new work is assigned. Instructional methods that require too much self-management of time on task do not work for these students.

Frequent evaluation to ensure learning is key to success working with this population. The approach used by the Morningside School program in Seattle, Washington, with children with NLD calls for daily evaluation of progress against expected outcomes. The program claims a high academic success rate, which it attributes mainly to careful and frequent measurement of results to guide acceleration of the topic or repetition of material.[135]

8. **Make extensive use of computerized teaching technology: A computer-friendly classroom is an AS- and HFA-friendly classroom.**

   Innovative computer technology makes learning more efficient for children with HFA and AS. Here are some basic accommodations:

   - If a child has problems with note taking and handwriting, a laptop computer or similar device should be assigned to her by the school district.

   - If lack of self-organization is a barrier to learning, the laptop should be programmed with all class work for the term or school year. This includes all lectures, requirements, and homework.

   - If following the teacher's auditory input is difficult, equip the child with software for her laptop that automatically scribes the teacher's instructional notes on the "board" (the teacher's laptop projected on the wall with LCD technology and PowerPoint software). These new devices, called "interactive whiteboards," replace the need for a student to have a personal scribe to capture notes, visuals, and multimedia for learning. This modification is an important asset to AS and HFA children who may have serious problems with short-term memory, auditory processing, and note taking.

## Conclusion: Help Children with HFA and AS Realize Their Gifts

The common gift of children with HFA and AS is the ability to visualize beauty in perfect form and function and to construct systems based on that vision. Children in these neurotypes are interested in the minutiae of how things work and they are able to put white-hot focus on the function of something to make it work better.

World culture is currently imperiled. Our climate is changing, our environment is polluted, and we are losing animal species. The United States and many other countries are involved in war. Violence and pandemic are upon us. New answers are needed. The ancient Celts said that when things were grim for a people, when crisis was at hand and nothing seemed to be working, "the Wyrd" would come to the fore. This term was used to describe all the mythic dwarves, strange and odd characters, who had the answers. The Celts knew that you had to be out of the mainstream to see the problem clearly. Michael Meade, a mythologist, says this about the Wyrd or weirdness in people in general:

> Each companion (figures in mythology with strange pow-
> ers) embodies capacities and powers beyond the normal.
> Each represents a connection to the wyrd – that is, to fate
> and destiny. Young people quickly perceive any essential
> strangeness in a person and label it "weird." To the young,
> this quality is both attractive and repulsive. It is often the
> actual point around which friendship forms, the place where
> the friends are connected … It is the weird parts of people
> that make unusual contributions to life. Denying the strange
> extremes and the deeply different aspects of people can turn
> their strangeness into something damaging to themselves
> and others. For the strangeness does not leave a person; it
> always finds a way to live itself out. Later in life, deeper in
> life, the "weirdness" in one person can help another move
> closer to his or her purpose and can remind each of a shared
> meaning in life. On a cultural level, what is incurable in one
> culture can often be healed by a weird or extreme aspect of
> another culture. Culturally diverse societies can find heal-
> ing in the variety of medicines carried inside the traditions
> of original cultures. In this way, multiplicity can unite what
> has been separate, and the "weird" can offer cures.[136]

Though I have no research to the effect, it is interesting to consider the possibility that the gene pool has created people capable of extreme effectiveness (truly Wyrd) to help the human race survive in this century. It is not impossible to consider that people with the gifts of technological genius of AS and the intense, unconventional creativity of HFA are among us in such great numbers because we need them to survive.

The first step is to recognize these children at home and in school. The second is to come up with realistic ways to make their lives successful and full. I hope, this chapter has been useful with regard to these two tasks. Our basic task as caregivers is to actively listen for the presence of each child's Great Story, his personal autobiography, and to build a foundation for achieving the child's destiny, regardless of how exalted or humble it may be. We may not know what his genius "wants" from him but we do know that creating the space for him to release it is the right thing to do.

## I Have A Fork
### by Joanne Barrie Lynn*

In order to help a child you must see the world through his eyes. This story is written from the perspective of James, an 8-year-old diagnosed with HFA. It provides a unique view of how children with autism think as well as how they perceive others. In highlighting the special gifts James possesses, it contrasts him with his sister, Jenny, a brilliant 6-year-old with AS. You may see that many of the traits and characteristics I described in Chapter One for AS and in Chapter Six for HFA are included in the narrative of the lives of James and Jenny. GTL

---

School is less bad this year because Mr. Turner is the new vice principal and he does not tolerate bullying at Nikola Tesla Elementary. Mr. Turner also lets my sister Jenny eat lunch in the cafeteria with me, even though she only goes to school until 12:15 p.m. Jenny is 6. I am 8.

I don't want to go to school any more. Mr. Turner can't stop all the bullies and I don't like getting yelled at and hit. Plus Jenny is too little to get hit. I want Mother or Father to home school Jenny and me. Aunt Emma says home schooling is good for kids like us. Father already teaches me astronomy. Maybe Mother could teach me biology.

Aunt Emma, Mother's sister, is teaching me how to deal with bullies. She is teaching me to do accessing, which is the same as remembering. She taught me to access a past success when I was bullied. The first time I did accessing, I couldn't think of a past success, so Aunt Emma said to think of someone big and strong and think what that person would do if he got bul-

*Joanne Barrie Lynn is a stress management and wellness educator, natural wood sculptor, and award-winning writer and poet whose work has been published in magazines, literary journals, and anthologies.*

lied. I thought of John Wayne, who is one of my heroes because he stands up to bullies and protects the weak, and because he has a weapon and he is not afraid to use it. The weapon is his Colt 44. He makes a fist around it with his thumb up and points it at the bully, and the bully loses the fight. Aunt Emma is also teaching me the Comedy Routine, where I think of funny things about the bully and laugh at him and give him a silly name. Like Bullet Head or Leather Jacket. Bullet Head and Leather Jacket are Jason Greene and Eliot Simpson. They are in sixth grade and push me in the halls and grab my backpack and yell at me. I don't know what they are saying because I can't understand when someone yells at me. The words all melt together. I'm not good at doing the Comedy Routine but Aunt Emma says that I will improve with age.

When Jenny eats lunch with me, she walks around the school after she gets out of her class. She counts her steps. At 12:27 p.m. she walks into the cafeteria. I save half my cookies for her. I like to eat lunch with Jenny. She walks home as soon as she has eaten her cookies. She counts her steps home.

Jenny has special needs. I do, too. I am dx HFA and Jenny is dx AS. Dx means diagnosed. HFA is the short way of saying high-functioning autism. AS is Asperger Syndrome. Grandpa Jimmy says AS is another kind of autism but he is wrong. HFA and AS are different.

Mother says I am HFA because I focus on everything around me instead of paying attention to one thing at a time, as if I'm walking around with my eyes very wide open, seeing everything all at once but not focused on anything. Mother says when I can't focus on one thing in particular, I have to learn everything all at once, and if you change one thing in the pattern I lose all of the pattern. Such as when Uncle Ben was teaching me how to bat and he said, "Remember the sweet spot." Uncle Ben always says that when I am at bat. It means remember to hit the ball on the exact spot on the bat that will exercise maximum force on the ball and hit it very far. On Saturday, September 10, at 1:35 p.m., Uncle Ben forgot to say the words and I couldn't swing the bat and I had a meltdown. Mother told me I had the meltdown because I have HFA. She said if I didn't have HFA I could swing the bat without Uncle Ben saying, "Remember the sweet spot," and I could remember the pattern even if one piece of it is missing.

Mother says I think in pictures because I am dx HFA. Grammie says I am a good translator from my pictures into words though I am not a chatterbox like my sister. Jenny thinks in words and numbers and likes to tell them to me all the time. Mother sings to Jenny when Jenny talks too much. "Amazing Voice How Sweet the Sound" is Jenny's favorite song and she always stops talking to listen.

Jenny does her math the same way I do my math. She sees the whole pattern in her mind and then finds the answer in it. I'm learning how to show my work, which means I write down all the steps through the pattern. That way Ms. Grierson, my math teacher, can see how I get to the answer. Ms. Grierson needs all the steps. She can't do math like us.

I went to the zoo with Father on Saturday, September 17, at 1:30 p.m. Father and I left Uncle Ben and my cousin Mark with the elephants and took the Northern Trail, stalking cougars. We didn't see any because cougars are nocturnal and solitary. At 7:32 p.m. we drove around Lake Washington to Juanita Bay Park and checked the wild beaver lodges. Beavers are most active at dusk and dawn; they are a keystone species because they are architects that change their habitat almost as much as humans, and we can learn from them. Uncle Ben is an architect and he likes the efficiency of entry and egress in a beaver lodge but not the blind sight lines. Mark likes them because they have no windows. I like the underwater entrance even though I can't see it. I can see the picture in my head because I saw the underwater doors in the beaver exhibit at Northwest Trek on Saturday, July 9, at 2:40 p.m. I saw a beaver dive down into the door and swim underwater across the pond in front of the window where people stand to watch them. Then he squeezed up into another lodge through the underwater entrance. Or she. Males and females are approximately the same size and have no visible distinguishing characteristics. They live in close proximity all winter in the dry dome part of the lodge and eat branches. They cut the branches with their incisors and float them to the lodge and store them underwater for the winter. Father says beavers mate for life and live harmoniously with their kits until they are grown up. Beaver lodges are my favorite houses. Father says beavers are my special interest, which means they are my favorite thought.

My favorite toy is two pairs of tiny sparkle shoes from Jenny's birthday cake, black and pink plastic. Black and pink are Jenny's favorite colors. My favorite colors are sparkles. I put the shoes in a patch of sun on the living room rug and move my head back and forth to watch the sparkles. I see pictures in sparkles. Jenny likes to talk to me when I look at the sparkle shoes.

Sometimes when I get too anxious, I can't think and I am very frustrated, so I scream and that helps. When Jenny gets too anxious, she has a meltdown. On Monday, September 19, at 4:36 p.m., Jenny threw Mother's favorite wedding vase onto the part of the living room floor where there is no rug and the wood is hard. Mother cried and swept up the broken pieces. Jenny screamed for 19 minutes.

Father and Mother bought Ramón the Robot for Jenny's birthday. On Sunday, September 11, at 3:13 p.m., Jenny made Ramón talk. Uncle Ben and Grandpa Jimmy laughed. Grammie said Ramón sounds exactly like Dustin Hoffman in *Rainman* and Father said even our robots are autistic. Jenny likes to build robots out of used computer parts. Father says robots are Jenny's special interest. She doesn't play with Ramón any more because she took him apart to make him walk faster and his legs stopped moving.

I like to draw the pictures that are in my head. I also draw what I see with my eyes, like the outside of beaver lodges. When I have an anxious moment, I draw small pictures. Father calls this doodling. He doodles too, but not as much as I do. Doodling is a self-calming activity and it helps me not scream. I have a small notebook and a tiny pencil in my pocket for doodling. The pencil is a golfer's pencil and is 6 centimeters long.

When I don't need to doodle, I draw with an ebony pencil in my sketchbook. I like to draw on slightly rough paper because I like how the pencil drags across it and because I can smudge shadows on it. I like to draw Jenny. She doesn't sit still very long, but I can draw her because I have so many Jenny pictures in my head. When she is reading or doing math she is still except for her hands and her tongue, which rubs the corners of her mouth. When she is thinking or frustrated, her left hand pats the desk or turns into a fist and thumps.

On Wednesday, September 14, at 10:37 a.m., I drew Jenny's fist thumping, and it turned into seven fists in seven slightly different positions above the desk. Ms. Osbourne, my art teacher, said that picture reminds her of a famous painting by Marcel Duchamps, who is a dead French Impressionist. She found the picture on the Internet and showed it to me. It is called Nude Descending a Staircase, and there is nothing in it that looks like a fist at all. But Ms. Osbourne said to look at the motion that the artist shows, and then I could see what she meant. On Friday, September 16, at 8:11 p.m., I tried to draw my sister during a meltdown, but she moved too fast and hard. Plus I don't like to be around her during a meltdown. She screams and that hurts my ears.

I read better than most college students. That is what the principal, Mrs. McLendon, told Father and Mother on Tuesday, August 30, at 11:51 a.m. She said that I read technical books about my special interests; I range from architectural structures to statistics of future habitats to bioethics and desertification. Father says we are an entire family of odd ducks and voracious readers, which means hungry. Father's favorite family evening is Starbucks and Half Price Books in Crossroads Mall, which is in Bellevue, Washington, and is 13.1 miles from our house. On Friday, September 23 at 7:12 p.m., I bought *Teach Your Own* by John Holt and told Mother and Father that I want them to homeschool Jenny and me. Then we got coffees and hot chocolates and listened to Father's friend Randy play jazz trombone on the Market Stage.

On Saturday, September 24, at 12:14 a.m., Mother told Father that she is already at her wit's end, and Father said Jenny needs the social involvement of regular school but why not turn the dining room into James' schoolroom. Mother said, over my dead body, don't I have enough to keep track of already with this autistic genius without trying to homeschool him too, for God's sake, when my major was vocal performance and my put-on-hold-forever career never came close to teaching. Father said it's not rocket science to teach history and biology to an 8-year-old and we can outsource the math.

I heard them when I got up to go pee and they were drinking wine by the fireplace and listening to one of Mother's CDs that she recorded before I was born. I used to do head-banging to self-calm. Mother says I did head-banging more than anyone she knows. Mother still tries to get me to wear my bike helmet all the time but I only wear it when I ride my bike. Jenny can't ride her bike. She can't get her balance right. Father says not to worry; she'll learn it in time. Mother says Jenny's balance is completely off, can't you see that darling Jenny isn't like James she's not autistic; she's a clumsy Asperger's, why can't you ever see that. Then they have a private discussion in their bedroom.

I still do screaming but only at home. I always try to give Mother and Father a warning first, because screaming makes them jump inside their bodies and is a danger signal, except for Jenny, who screams for small things, like tripping on a tool. I don't scream as much as Jenny.

I don't do head-banging any more. I stopped on Wednesday, August 17, at 10:14 a.m. because Dr. Paul, our family physician, drew me a diagram of the brain to show me what head-banging does to the prefrontal cortex. He said that if I do head-banging I will eventually lose my thinking. He gave me the brain diagram. Mother stuck it on the fridge with my four beaver magnets. I don't want to lose my thinking.

I consulted Dr. Paul on Wednesday, August 31, at 11:27 a.m., about Jenny's screaming. Dr. Paul said that I am a good brother to Jenny and that it is the job of the adults in Jenny's life, like him and Mother and Father, to take care of Jenny; my job is to grow up smart and strong. Then Dr. Paul told Mother that Jenny's screaming is caused by her high level of anxiety and won't hurt anything but our ears, and that a medication that raises her serotonin levels might help, like maybe Lexapro, which is a Selective Serotonin Reuptake Inhibitor that would help Jenny's brain calm down, so why not make an appointment with Dr. Wilson.

On Wednesday, September 28, which is today, when Jenny counted steps into the cafeteria to eat lunch with me at 12:27 p.m., Bullet Head and Leather Jacket saw her, and they yelled and tried to grab her. Jenny is fast, so she got away from them and sat down next to me and started to eat her cookies. Bullet Head and Leather Jacket yelled the bully words and ran around the table to get Jenny.

So I did accessing like Aunt Emma taught me. I remembered John Wayne. I stood up and made my sister get behind me. I found a weapon. It was my fork. I made a fist around it like John Wayne. I pointed it at Bullet Head and looked at the space between his eyebrows and said I have a fork and I'm not afraid to use it. Bullet Head made a squeaky noise and looked at Leather Jacket. Then Mr. Turner was there and he put his hand on my shoulder and said, hold on there, cowboy and told Bullet Head and Leather Jacket to go to his office and wait for him. He would deal with them there.

Mr. Turner explained that I can't threaten anyone with a weapon again, even a plastic fork, or I will be expelled. I explained to Mr. Turner that I have to protect my sister. Then I holstered my fork in my pocket.

Mother drove us both home even though I was supposed to go to math. She said I was very brave to protect Jenny but I shouldn't have to deal with bullies and it's up to the adults to see that bullying doesn't happen. Then she pounded her right fist on the steering wheel. She looked like Jenny except Jenny pounds her left fist. Mother said Damn that Emma!

## Deconstructing Autism: A Summary of Features of James' Character as a Child with High-Functioning Autism

| Narrative from the Story | Comment |
| --- | --- |
| "Aunt Emma is teaching me to do accessing." And "Aunt Emma is also teaching me the Comedy Routine." | Children with autism and AS benefit from learning, by rote, concrete, visual and auditory prompts to help them in stressful situations. Many children with HFA are very accomplished mimics and have acting potential. The late master actor Peter Sellers is probably one good example. |
| "They are in sixth grade and push me in the halls and grab my backpack and yell at me. I don't know what they are saying because I can't understand when someone yells at me." | Sensory overload may cause impairment in cognitive function in children with HFA, who are primary targets for every bully at school. |
| "When Jenny eats lunch with me, she walks around the school after she gets out of her class. She counts her steps. At 12:27 p.m. she walks into the cafeteria." | As is the case for many kids with AS, Jenny is very precise and somewhat obsessive. She has developed a system to "wire around" her fixed-figure perceptual style. |
| "Mother says I am HFA because I focus on everything around me instead of paying attention to one thing at a time, as if I'm walking around with my eyes very wide open, not focused on anything in particular. Mother says because I can't focus on anything in particular I have to learn everything all at once, and if you change one thing in the pattern I go ballistic." | Here James explains the idea that people with autism take in everything in their perceptual environment at once. This is what I call a full-field perceptual style. They see everything as background and cannot focus on individual objects against the ground or easily move from focusing on one discrete object to another. |
| "Mother says I think in pictures because I am dx HFA." | Children with HFA have powerful mental visual processing skills and test higher on visual IQ subtests. |

**Deconstructing Autism: A Summary of Features of James' Character as a Child with High-Functioning Autism (continued)**

| Narrative from the Story | Comment |
|---|---|
| "Jenny does her math the same way I do my math." | Many children with HFA and AS have superior math skills for different reasons. AS children use their powerful verbal abilities for remembering, categorizing, computing, and listing. HFA children may use visual algorithms or visual-intuitive devices such as Einstein's statement that he came to his famous equation $E=MC^2$ "riding on a beam of light." |
| "I like the underwater entrance even though I can't see it. I can see the picture in my head because I saw the underwater doors in the beaver exhibit at Northwest Trek on Saturday, July 9, at 2:40 p.m." | HFA children are powerful visual processors. The great inventor Nikola Tesla, a probable autistic, calmed his mind as a boy so he could sleep by visualizing his inventions in operation from above, below, and on all sides. |
| "My favorite toy is two pairs of tiny sparkle shoes from Jenny's birthday cake, black and pink plastic. Black and pink are Jenny's favorite colors. My favorite colors are sparkles. I put the shoes in a patch of sun on the living room rug and move my head back and forth to watch the sparkles. I see pictures in sparkles." | Autistic children tend to be fascinated by the details of things. True to the narrative of people like Temple Grandin, they tend to seek perfect visual beauty. |
| "When Jenny gets too anxious, she has a meltdown. On Monday, September 19, at 4:36 p.m. Jenny threw Mother's favorite wedding vase onto the part of the living room floor where there is no rug and the wood is hard. Mother cried and swept up the broken pieces. Jenny screamed for 19 minutes." | This is a good description of a meltdown. If rage were the issue, Jenny would behave much more violently. There would be much greater pathos in the scene. HFA kids report to me that they self-soothe with screaming and AS kids often say that a meltdown helps them release frustration. |

**Deconstructing Autism: A Summary of Features of James' Character
as a Child with High-Functioning Autism (continued)**

| Narrative from the Story | Comment |
|---|---|
| "I like to draw Jenny. She doesn't sit still very long, but I can draw her because I have so many Jenny pictures in my head. When she is reading or doing math she is still except for her hands and her tongue, which rubs the corners of her mouth." | This illustrates James' ability from his full-field perceptual style to record and process images in his field in precise detail.<br><br>The visual perceptual style of people with autism is discussed by Dr. Oliver Sacks in his description of British artist Steven Wiltshire.[137] |
| "I drew Jenny's fist thumping, and it turned into seven fists in seven slightly different positions above the desk. Ms. Osbourne, my art teacher, said that picture reminds her of a famous painting by Marcel Duchamps, who is a dead French Impressionist." | |
| "I used to do head-banging to self-calm." "I still do screaming but only at home." | Some HFA children report that their disturbing behavior has a very specific self-soothing function. |
| "Jenny can't ride her bike. She can't get her balance right. Father says not to worry; she'll learn it in time. Mother says, "Jenny's balance is completely off, can't you see that darling Jenny isn't like James? She's not autistic; she's a clumsy Asperger's, why can't you ever see that?" | AS problems with left-right coordination are very common. They are much less common in HFA kids, who may be quite coordinated as youngsters but become very ungainly as teens. |
| "My favorite toy is two pairs of tiny sparkle shoes." | Many children with autism are fascinated by shiny objects and derive joy from staring at them. This is also mentioned in the Appendix of autistic writer Donna Williams' book *Nobody Nowhere*.[138] From my observation of my clients I believe that this feature is not seen as often in children diagnosed with AS. |

## Deconstructing Autism: A Summary of Features of James' Character as a Child with High-Functioning Autism (continued)

| Narrative from the Story | Comment |
| --- | --- |
| "Doodling is a self-calming activity and helps me not scream." | Drawing is a calming practice for many children with HFA. |
| "I pointed it at Bullet Head and looked at the space between his eyebrows and said 'I have a fork and I'm not afraid to use it.'" | In this event, James uses an imaginative Social Story™ to provide a program of action in a high stress situation. He is able, in true HFA fashion, to "get lost" in his character and, visually remembering its manner, let it guide his actions. |

## Endnotes

109. Wing, 1993.
110. Prince-Hughes, 2004.
111. Ishisaka, Y. et al. (1997). Cognitive deficits of autism based on results of three psychological tests. *Japanese Journal of Child and Adolescent Psychiatry, 38*(3), 230-246. (This study suggests that children with autism have difficulty integrating meaning from the Rorschach test that includes "cognition of the structure of a situation" – how it fits into its background.)
112. Bogdashina, O. (2003). (Accessed August 2005). *Different sensory experiences-different sensory worlds.* www.autismtoday.com/articles/Different_Sensory_Experiences.htm
113. Rinehart, 2002. p. 326.
114. *Diagnostic and statistical manual IV*; Baron-Cohen S., & Gilberg, C. (1992). Can autism be detected at 18 months? The needle, the haystack, and the CHAT. *British Journal of Psychiatry, 161*, 839; National Institute of Mental Health. (2004, April). *Autism spectrum disorders* (Information Pamphlet, NIH Publication No. 04-5511); American Psychiatric Association, 2000.
115. (for eye movement thinking style assessment): Bandler, R., & Grinder, J. (1979). *Frogs into princes.* Moab, UT: Real People Press. p. 25.
116. Grandin, T. (Accessed 2005). *My experiences with visual thinking sensory problems and communication difficulties.* Center for the Study of Autism. http://www.autism.org/temple/visual.html.
117. Williams, 1992. p. 211.
118. Siegel, 1999. p. 36.

119. Gray, C. (1994). *Comic strip conversations*. Arlington, TX: Future Horizons; Myles, B. S. (2001). Using social stories and comic strip conversations to interpret social situations for an adolescent with Asperger Syndrome. *Intervention in School and Clinic, 36*(5), 310.

120. Lynn, 2000.

121. Grandin, 1995. p. 192.

122. Sabbagh, M. (2004, June). p. 209. Dr. Sabbagh and colleagues point to underdevelopment of the orbitofrontal cortex as the culprit involved in the problem that people on the autistic spectrum have with emotional decoding; Baron-Cohen, S. et al. (2000, May). The amygdala theory of autism. *Neuroscience and Behavioral Reviews, 24*(3), 355-364.

123. Hindman, J. (1983). *A very touching book*. Baker City, OR: Alexandria Associates.

124. Reiner, 2003. p. 24.

125. Hillman, J. (1996) *The soul's code: In search of character and calling*. New York: Random House. p. 17; Barnhill, G., Hagiwara, T., Myles, B. S., & Simpson, R. L. (2000). Asperger Syndrome: A study of the cognitive profiles of 37 children and adolescents. *Focus on Autism and Other Developmental Disabilities, 15*(3), 146-153.

126. Minshew, N. et al. (1997). Neuropsychologic functioning in autism: Profiles of a complex information processing disorder. *Journal of the International Neuropsychological Society, 3*(4), 303-316.

127. Goldstein, G. et al. (2001). A comparison of WAIS-R profiles in adults with high-functioning autism or differing subtypes of learning disability. *Applied Neuropsychology, 8*(13), 148-154.

128. Ishisaka, 1997. p. 230.

129. Goldstein, 2001. p.148.

130. Mayes, S. D. (2003). Ability profiles in children with autism: Influence of age and IQ. *Autism, 7*(1), 65-80.

131. Mayes, S. D. et al. (2004). Similarities and differences in Wechsler Intelligence Scale for Children – Third Edition. *Clinical Neuropsychologist, 18*(4), 559-572.

132. This list includes items developed by Dr. Temple Grandin. Grandin, T. (Accessed 2005). *Teaching tips for children and adults with autism*. Center for the Study of Autism. http://www.autism.org/temple/tips.html

133. Nelson, L. (2001). (Accessed September 2005). *Communication strategies for adults with autistic spectrum disorders*. http://www.SpeechSense.com

134. Kluth, P. (Accessed October 2005). *A supportive communication partner*. http://www.paulakluth.com

135. Johnson & Layng, 1992.

136. Meade, M. (1993). *Men and the water of life*. San Francisco: Harper. p. 387.

137. Sacks, O. (1995). *An anthropologist on mars*. New York: Knopf.

138. Williams, 1992.

Chapter Seven

# How to Help the Child with Asperger Syndrome also Diagnosed with Tourette's Syndrome

Tourette's syndrome (TS) is a neurological disorder in which a person makes repetitive vocalizations such as snorts, grunts, barks, hoots, or obscene words, and repetitive muscle movements such as eye blinking, head throwing, kicking, or grimacing. These repetitive movements and sounds are called "tics." In order to qualify for the diagnosis of TS, both motor and vocal tics must be present, although not necessarily at the same time. In addition, these tics must have been present for over a year and not be ascribed to any other disorder. Children who have tics report that the tics are often preceded by feelings in the musculature, described as a "muscle itch," to do something that compels the tic to occur. These are called "premonitory" sensations and are relieved by performance of the tic only to reoccur soon after. Tics typically "wax and wane." That is, a child may suffer from a certain tic for a week, a month, or a year, but then it will disappear only to be replaced by another tic.

People with TS are also said to suffer from "perseverative behaviors." That is, they repeat words and actions and/or mimic the words and actions of others. Some of the ways that the tendency toward perseverance is expressed include echolalia (repeating what others have just said), echopraxia (mimicking others' actions), coprolalia (swearing or using vulgar words), coprographia (writing dirty words), and copropraxia (using sexually inappropriate gestures). Children diagnosed with TS display unusual creativity, combining these behaviors.[139]

Perseverative behaviors are also expressed in obsessive thoughts and compulsive behavior. Obsessions and compulsions (OC) occur very frequently in children with TS although not in all. Obsessions and compulsions occur very frequently among children diagnosed with AS. Chapter Four provided strategies for managing the challenge of OC in AS kids at home and at school so I will not go into detail on the subject in this chapter. The best strategies manage the symptoms of OC regardless of co-existing diagnoses. I advise parents to do the same things to help their obsessing children whether their kids are diagnosed with AS or TS.

About a third of the children I work with who are diagnosed with TS have a robust "potty humor." This complex coprolalia is manifested by talking about farting, toilet use, and all things scatological. They delight in talking about excrement, and enjoy hooking adults into scolding them for talking about these subjects. Given the prominence of the limbic brain in the personality of the Tourettic child, it makes sense that he should express the animality of his nature with themes involving all the bodily functions.

Some researchers believe Amadeus Mozart had TS with coprographia. Dr. Ruth Bruun, a neurologist with a specialty in TS, has found many examples of coprographic-like text in Mozart's writing. Here is one such quoted in her book *A Mind of Its Own: Tourette's Syndrome, A Story and a Guide.* From one of his letters dated November 5, 1777:

> Dearest Coz Fuzz!
> I have received reprieved your dear letter telling, selling me that my uncle carbuncle, my aunt can't and you too are very well, hell …
> I am very sorry to heart that Abbott rabbit has had another stroke so soon moon. But I trust that with God's Cod's help it will have no serious consequences excrescences … I shit on your nose and it will run down your chin. (From letter number 236).[140]

## Children with Asperger Syndrome and Tourette's Syndrome

Many children with a primary diagnosis of AS or Autistic Disorder also have tics and meet the criteria for TS. One study revealed that 20% of children with a primary diagnosis of AS or HFA are eventually also diagnosed with TS.[141]

The DSM-IV defines "stereotypical mannerisms" to be the rocking, clapping, and toe walking seen in some cases of autism. However, the distinction between these phenomena and Tourettic tics is unclear. What, for instance, is the difference in neurological etiology between a tic shown in a child's repetitive hand flapping from the elbow (as if to flick something off the end of his finger) and the elbows in the flapping gesture made by some children with autism? Though research is unclear on the point, the common denominator of the behavior is its perseverative nature – its tendency to repeat a movement. In autism, a child may get relief from anxiety for performing the movement. In TS, the child reports relief from the premonitory itch. In both situations, the movement serves to decrease unpleasant over-excitation in the form of anxiety and the urge to tic to relieve the itch.

My clinical experience confirms the presence of Tourettic phenomena in many children with a primary diagnosis of AS. I look for what I term the "trunk" neurotype when beginning work with a child. That is, I try to identify the diagnosis that most accurately describes the child's inner life and is fundamental to her personality and challenges. Other issues may accompany this basic neurotype but are secondary to it in terms of the focus for treatment.

Making an accurate trunk diagnosis between AS and TS is essential in my practice because if I do not deal directly with the child's most basic challenges, all my attempts to help him will miss the mark. Children with the stand-alone diagnosis of TS are very different neurologically and behaviorally from children with stand-alone AS, and each neurotype requires a different kind of help. In the social domain, for example, children with TS may have neurotypical social skills but be greatly bedeviled by a tendency to lose their tempers and be chronically combative. These are not necessarily issues commonly faced by kids with AS, who suffer more from the inability to make friends but may be able to keep them once a friendship is started. In brief, one neurotype needs help with anger management, the other with social pragmatics.

As noted above, children diagnosed with AS and those diagnosed with both AS and TS experience obsessions and compulsions. There is a lot of confusion as to whether a child's odd movement is a stereotyped motor mannerism or a compulsion.

Dr. Mort Duran is a neurosurgeon specializing in Tourette's syndrome who is Tourettic himself. According to Duran, children perform compulsions to achieve a sense of balance and "evening up." Tics, on the other hand, may be seen as movements in response to a feeling, the muscle itch known as a pre-monitory. Children are usually able to identify the origin of their behaviors as an OC or a tic using these criteria.[142]

## Tourette's Syndrome, Asperger Syndrome, or Both? Criteria for Determining an Accurate Trunk Diagnosis

Once the presence of tics is ascertained, the next step is to determine if a child is experiencing TS as a stand-alone condition or AS with features of TS.

To sort for the presence of AS, I look for the following signatory features. Please keep in mind that in the AS-plus-TS neurotype, AS always trumps TS. That is, the challenges that the child faces from AS are the challenges that will become the primary focus of attention.

1. **Does the child communicate emotionally?**

   The children I work with diagnosed with TS tend to be very emotional. They make intense eye contact and enjoy bantering and joking.

   Although there is little research on this aspect of TS, researchers do suggest that the limbic brain – the locus of a person's emotional life – is highly active in TS. This literature refers to the impulsivity, speed, joy in movement and rage of many people with TS. For example, commenting about rage in TS, Dr. Oliver Sacks writes: "Tourette's is like an epilepsy in the subcortex; when it takes over, there's just a thin line of control, a thin line of cortex between you and it, between you and that raging storm, the blind force of the subcortex."[143]

   Although I rarely see the foreboding rage, the striking out, that Dr. Sacks refers to, I do see the joy and the pain in these kids. That sense of "thin line" between them and their experience of the world is very real, and it is hard for them to hold back, to be polite, and to stifle what they have to say and not express what they feel.

   In contrast to the aggressive jocularity of the child with TS, the child with AS tends to be rather "wooden" in his interpersonal commu-nications. His voice tone may be flat and his language syntax is logi-cal, often quite thoughtful, but devoid of emotional charge. It is very difficult for him to engage in the give-and-take of argument, although he may enjoy debating and "negotiating" in a "logic-oriented way" (e.g., pseudologic). He may also be very good at directive pestering and whining to get things his way.

If a child shows a flat affect in his communications, I put a check-mark in my mind in the "possibly AS (or HFA)" column. For one reason or another, some children with TS demonstrate a flat emotional tone so I do not consider this a "necessary and sufficient" criterion for identification of AS, but still give it weight in my evaluation.

2. **What is his friend-making style? Does he have difficulty making friends (AS) or keeping them (TS)?**
   Children with TS and those with AS may or may not be successful in making friends. However, children with AS are somewhat disadvantaged socially because of a lack of social pragmatics and have difficulty initiating friendships. If a child's AS is mild, he may have passable social skills and be able to link up with one or two "best friends," who may show features of AS themselves.

   Children with TS, on the other hand, show neurotypical ability to make friends but may not keep them because they have difficulty controlling irritability and depressive affect. They may also tend to "jump boundaries" with friends, such as getting too close physically, having temper tantrums, or asking overly personal questions.

   These sort of difficulties are also seen in AS and HFA but have a different cause. In TS, boundary jumping and combativeness are related to the child's basic impulsivity. Unlike kids with AS or HFA who do not understand the concept of personal space or appropriate social conversation, the child with TS may well understand these factors but feel pushed by his hyper-energized nervous system to proceed anyway. "Impulsivity" and "compulsivity" are words that describe his issues in this regard. In AS and HFA, it is the lack of a certain cognitive set that hampers friend making; the inability to make good assumptions about others' intentions and needs.

3. **Is he typically combative or aversive when stressed? Is he effectively combative?**
   When children with HFA or AS are stressed, they typically take the "flight" path to managing the stress, and the meltdowns that they have when frustrated or overstressed tend to push others away. They are motivated by a desire for stimulus safety.[144]

Children with AS are not by nature aggressive. Most of the AS and HFA children I work with do not have good ability to sense another's move in a conflict and respond quickly and decisively. This may be a result of the difficulty that both neurotypes have in coordinating thought and movement rapidly. When they are "aggressive," they are typically trying to defend themselves. They are not good at offensively striking out to gain an advantage. At school, they are bullied. They rarely bully others. They can be annoying because of their character rigidity and obsessionality, but they are typically gentle by nature.

There is also a very high co-morbidity between TS, ADD, and ADD with AD/HD. The child who is TS plus AD/HD may display a powerful athletic intelligence and capacity for much energized play of any sport he chooses. For some reason, many TS boys enjoy wrestling. Perhaps it is their enjoyment of physical contact combined with the opportunity for aggressive encounter that brings them to this sport.

The child who is TS plus ADD (inattentive type) shows the presence of high creativity, often in the arts and sciences, but is not as outgoing. These children may be friendless because their tics are annoying or scary to other kids. This kind of social isolation is experienced as shaming and they withdraw into depressive affect. Indeed, this child is at some risk of developing depression because of his reflexive tendency to pull back into himself when stressed.

One research study of children with the dual diagnosis of AS and TS documented significant brain abnormalities in the children with AS that were not present in children with the stand-alone diagnosis of TS.[145] The cognitive challenges of AS trump the motor and vocal tics of TS. Though having tics may make a child's life miserable, it is the cognitive and social impairments that come with AS that make it the "trunk" diagnosis – the child's most profound disorder. That is why, if I am evaluating a child with tics, I look closely at the quality of his aggressive behavior, his impulsivity, and his athletic ability. Strong evidence of these factors argues against presence of AS. It is important to make this distinction because it is the cognitive and social impairments that will sabotage the child's life if they are not addressed. Longitudinal research[146] indicates that the tics may fade when the child grows into his twenties. AS does not lessen in intensity in this manner.

It is appropriate to offer a caveat when discussing the relative disadvantage children with AS have in athletics. That is, although they may not do well in fast-paced team sports, they may show excellence in solitary athletic forms such as the martial arts, which reward their ability to learn by repetition and practice certain stylized combat movements until they are second nature and delivered perfectly. Children with AS may do well at team sports but this is not the rule. Certainly, any AS child with a co-existing NLD will have difficulty making the rapid decisions in coordination with teammates required of any fast-paced team sport. But as is the case with children with HFA, practice makes perfect. Thus, AS children's capacity for intense focus gives them advanced ability to demonstrate perfect form in the martial arts, and their tendency to obsessionality ensures that every move will be well practiced.

## 4. What are his characterological strengths?

Children of both neurotypes show an interest in how systems work and possess gifts as inventors in the arts and sciences, with TS kids being inclined to artistic invention. As mentioned, according to Dr. Ruth Bruun, there is strong likelihood that Mozart had TS.[147]

In my experience, children with AS are more oriented toward mechanical-technical creativity and invention. Children of both neurotypes tend to disturb things. Be it the powerful persistence of an AS child in pursuit of her special interest or the taboo-breaking swearing of a child with TS, these children rock the boat. To quote the great systems theorist Ilya Prigogine, they provide the "disturbance" that all systems need to renew themselves and survive.[148] Possessing this characteristic, they are difficult to parent and difficult to reach in the classroom.

I have observed that children with TS, HFA, and AS have an affinity for music but their talents in this regard are somewhat different. Children with TS have a bent toward original music composition and are innovative and wildly creative players.

Children with HFA whom I have worked with do not typically show a flair for musical composition. There is too much writing involved. Though I do not have a large population sample, several of these HFA children do have a talent for exact replication of the playing style of other composers and musicians. They enjoy writing computer anime games and are brilliant synthesizers of different musical formats to accompany their anime creations. As mentioned, a review of the life of the great Bach interpreter Glenn Gould shows presence of the features of HFA, including the fact that he would not play for others, only for himself.

I have noticed strengths in technical music composition and play in the children I work with diagnosed with AS. As players, they may have excellent auditory discrimination and play a piece flawlessly as it was written. Music to most children with AS is not an opportunity for the expression of wild emotional and physical energy as it is for TS children. I theorize that children with AS are more likely to be teachers of musical composition than improvisers, and gravitate toward a particular way to express musical interest. Children with TS prefer the drums and the wild improvisation possible with this instrument. They have excellent kinesthetic (feeling-based) memory.

Children with TS also possess a powerful empathy with animals and the natural world. If I want to bridge conversation and form rapport with these kids, I talk about animals, how they think, and the way they are misunderstood. I get rapport right away.

My AS clients rarely describe enjoyment from witnessing natural beauty. Several are avid Boy Scouts and enjoy backpacking, hiking, and the opportunity for accomplishment afforded by being in Scouts. However, these are not the children who become awestruck by a beautiful sunset. To them, a beautiful sunset is "ho hum." More interesting are the scientific names and properties of floura and fauna seen on Scouting trips.

## 5. What are the child's learning challenges?

Children in each neurotype possess characteristic learning challenges. Although the possession of these LDs is in no way essential to the diagnosis, I have found it useful, in deciding if a child better fits the pattern of TS or AS, to take a good look at what kind of learning problems she experiences. This is especially important if the child also has an NLD. As noted in Chapter Three, some research indicates that about half of the kids diagnosed with AS also show presence of an NLD.[149]

While NLD is very common in AS, it is much less so in TS. If NLD is present, the AS child has difficulty forming abstractions from her experience and retaining learning from personal experience. And she will fear novelty. Paradoxically, the "Asperger mind" may be very good at solving problems in which there are known variables. This ability is related to the powerful auditory memory often seen in kids with AS.

My clinical experience suggests that the creative style of the child with TS is very different from the creative style of the child with AS. I observe that TS children tend to be very creative in a variety of artistic forms and possess a powerful "what if" type of inventive creativity. Not possessing the NLD-related problems in forming abstractions or working with unknown factors, their characterological nonconformity is an asset for looking at things from different perspectives and forming conclusions that would not occur to others.

Children with TS are more likely than children with AS to have learning problems like those seen in children with ADD – problems in "executive functions."

A co-existing ADD or ADHD has been found in a large number of children diagnosed with TS. These children typically carry the executive function problems characteristic of children with ADD and AD/HD. One researcher, Dr. David Comings, found that either AD/HD or ADD (inattentive type) was present in half the children in his study population who were diagnosed with TS.[150]

These issues include problems paying attention, short-term memory, getting started on things, and avoiding distraction. Although problems with executive function may be seen in children properly diagnosed with AS, AS kids tend to have excellent memory for detail and, once begun on a project, they are more likely to experience problems with hyperfocus than with distractibility.

## Major Characteristics of Children with TS vs. AS

| Domain of Function | Tourette's Syndrome | Asperger Syndrome |
|---|---|---|
| 1. Communication style | Highly emotional verbal and nonverbal behavior. | Highly logical verbal behavior; diminished nonverbal expression. |
| 2. Friend-making style | Makes friends but cannot keep them because of impulsivity and social aggressiveness. | Difficulty making friends. If successful, keeps them. |
| 3. Conflict response style | • Combative, counterdependent, aggressive; or<br><br>• Somewhat withdrawn and conflict avoidant. (Mirroring the AD/HD vs. ADD distinction.) | • Aversive and passive.<br><br>• Low skilled in physical combat, clumsy.<br><br>• May be able to master a martial art in which "practice makes perfect." |
| 4. Character strengths | • Interested in how systems work – "system disturbers."<br><br>• Artistic and musical inventor.<br><br>• Plays well by ear; enjoys improvisation (drums).<br><br>• Excellent kinesthetic and auditory memory.<br><br>• Finds beauty in nature.<br><br>• Fast, in sports or fights with other kids. | • Interested in how systems work – "system disturbers."<br><br>• Scientific and technical inventor.<br><br>• Teaches music, enjoys perfection of score.<br><br>• Excellent auditory memory.<br><br>• Finds beauty in seamless function of machines and systems. |
| 5. Learning disabilities | • May be excellent creative thinker but lack good "executive function" and shows LDs typical of ADD. | Nonverbal learning problems: Does not do well with open-ended problems and formation of abstractions. |

## Key Strategies for Helping the AS-Plus-TS Child at Home and at School

1. **Teach the child to use natural habit reversal (NHR) to reduce his tics.**
   Research indicates that tics may be decreased or eliminated by deliberately resisting the urge to tic while performing a substitute behavior. This method, called "habit reversal,"[151] has been shown to change brain function so as to permanently heal the errant neurological reaction that produces tics. The habit reversal protocol, when formally conducted in a treatment setting such as a psychologist's office, includes four steps:

   - *Awareness.* The child is taught to recognize the premonitory feelings in her musculature that precede the urge to tic.

   - *Relaxation.* The child practices breathing or other techniques to calm herself neurologically.

   - *Competing response.* The child refuses the urge to tic or executes a different movement. For example, if she has the urge to throw her head quickly to the right, as she experiences the premonition feeling, she leans very slowly to the left. Competing responses must be crafted individually for children based on how they describe a particular urge to tic.

   - *Positive cognitive focus.* (This step is also called "contingency management.") The child is encouraged to keep a positive vision of how her future will improve once she has worked through the tics she experiences.

   In a clinical procedure, the child would be scheduled to practice these steps every day for six weeks for a certain period of time, helped by a parent or coach. I rarely encounter children challenged by tics who have the energy or willingness to go through this protocol, so I advise the use of what I term natural habit reversal (NHR) – to use a competing response unobtrusively whenever and wherever they can do so. This approach has been used successfully with a number of the Tourettic children and adolescents I have worked with.

   Using NHR, a child experiencing an eye-blink tic can interrupt the tic and eventually extinguish it by palming his eyes when he gets the premonitory to tic. I suggest that the child apply light pressure from the palms of the hands to his closed eyes while imagining something very dark, such as outer space or black fur. Another example of NHR involves reversal of a head-throw tic. Upon getting the premonitory to tic, the child refrains from doing the tic and instead gently massages his neck while rotating his head slowly in a direction counter to the tic. This is a commonly used stress management technique. I have found that kids can be very creative in coming up with competing responses that fit them.

2.  **Help the child formulate what to say to other kids about his tics.**
    The population of children who experience tics is divided into two groups: Those who are O.K. with telling people about their condition and those who are mortified by having tics and loathe to discuss them. Regardless of the child's comfort level with disclosing information about her tics, it is important that she have a way of explaining them to other children. If she does not, she runs the risk of being isolated for being "weird" or "mental." I advocate the use of Mitchell Vitiello's approach, described in the book written by people with Tourette's entitled *Don't Think About Monkeys*.[152]

    Vitiello had the breakthrough awareness about his tics as a child in elementary school that if they did not matter to him, they did not seem to matter to anyone else. Using this tact, work with the child to give him as much acceptance of his tics as he would being near-sighted or having a bothersome cold. Let him know that if he can move past being self-conscious, things will change for the better. And, teach him verbal strategies to move this process along. For example, when asked by another child about his tics, teach him to say things like:

    1.  "Don't worry. I'm not contagious."

    2.  "They're just my tics."

    3.  "I have a neurological condition."

    4.  "I have Tourette's syndrome."

    5.  "Those are just my movements. I have to make them."

    As the child becomes more accepting of the TS aspects of his character (whether his tics are accompanied by features of AS or not), he is able to relax his painful self-consciousness around his tics. And as his anxiety decreases, his self-defeating social behaviors and learning problems lessen. It makes sense to pay attention to his feelings around having tics so as to draw him out and help him develop personal re-sourcefulness to deal with the all-important social dimension.

3.  **Include the child on her IEP team.**
    If a child is old enough and capable of following the discussion of her IEP team and answer questions, she should be included in its meetings. If she is, it is important that all the adults present follow the rule of "describe behavior only." This means that in talking about the child's deportment at school, they do not make personal references to her char-acter but stick to describing what she does or does not do that gets in the way of her success. For example, they do not say, "You are ticcing just for the attention and special treatment it gets you." "You can't help what you are doing because you have obsessive compulsive disorder." Or "You are just lazy. You could do the work if you wanted to." These kinds of statements indict the child's personality, her being, and do not point her toward things she can do to change. More important, these sort of comments shame; they make who she is (not what she does) the problem.

    Describing behavior does not shame the child. For example, an adult might say (instead of blaming the child for attention seeking), "You seem to tic more when you get stressed in class. How can we help reduce your stress?" Or, instead of criticizing him for being "ob-sessive," "You are talking too much about your special interest (bugs) and that is disturbing the class. I need to ask you to write down your questions and put them in my in-basket. I will get back to you during your study skills period to answer them." Or, instead of calling him lazy, "You have not turned in much of your homework this term. What is the problem with that from your perspective and how can we help?"

    It is important for the child to be present because only he can de-scribe how the experience of tics affects academic performance. In Chapter Seven of *Survival Strategies for Parenting Children with Bi-polar Disorder*,[153] I suggested that many children with TS are perfectly happy having tics and value them as ways to improve focus. These kids have told me that when they are ticcing, they are focusing. When they are repressing the urge to tic, they cannot focus. The reality that not all children who experience them perceive tics as a symptom of illness underlines the importance of talking with the child before devising any academic accommodation. Any IEP-devised intervention should provide genuine help to the child. If the team devises a behavior plan that calls for the child's removal from class whenever he tics, he is being deprived of his education and may react to the injustice with vigorous oppositionality.

4. **Normalize the child's presence in the class.**
What the human mind does not understand, it fears. To diminish the fear caused by the ticcing child's behavior, spend some time telling the other students in the room about the various kinds of neuropsychiatric and physical disabilities children have. Talk about ADD, TS, and AS, and make it clear that kids with these conditions are not "doing it to get attention." Let them know that children with these issues want the same thing that every kid wants – to succeed in school and have friends. Then talk about how each of these conditions interferes with friend making.

Model total acceptance of the child's motor and vocal tics using a matter-of-fact tone. Give the child discretion to leave the room and resort to the "refuge" room provided by the school to express his tics. Remember, some children troubled by tics focus better when they are ticcing. Thus, staying in class may be the least restrictive environment for the child.

The primary challenge for most children with TS as a stand-alone condition is obsessionality. A tendency to perseverate is also found in the neurotype of AS. If a child is challenged by AS and also has tics, there is a high probability that she suffers from obsessions. Be on the lookout for these "silent saboteurs" of the child's progress and build rapport with her to work on devising ways for her to get her work done in class despite her obsessive mind-chatter. Children will hide their obsessions, so the best way to gain rapport is matter-of-fact talking from your own experience and observation.

**5. Write a behavior management plan that is part of the solution.**

A behavior management plan written for the AS-plus-TS child should not just help control the child's behavior, but should contribute to his education. It should help him develop the ability to make choices and take care of himself. In Chapter Two, I provided details of a behavior management plan for children with the AS-plus-BD neurotype. Core elements of these plans are similar, but actions to be taken by school staff are quite dissimilar.

The table below contains examples of the kinds of information that would be contained in a behavior plan written for an AS child challenged by motor and vocal tics and OCs in class.

**Key Aspects of a Behavior Plan for an AS Child with TS Tics**

| 1. Identify his character strengths. | • Enjoys competing with other kids in sports and academic contests.<br>• Excels in martial arts and track.<br>• Shows willingness to take risks such as speaking in front of the class.<br>• Has demonstrated personal honesty and sense of justice and generosity.<br>• Enjoys playful verbal bantering with other children. |
|---|---|
| 2. Identify his challenges. | • May be combative and oppositional short of meltdown or rage.<br>• May refuse to follow instructions and get argumentative with his teachers.<br>• May not show understanding of the informal rules of play.<br>• May seek excessive perfection in his work and will not turn something in if less than perfect.<br>• May demonstrate ADD-related executive function problems and is very poorly organized most of the time.<br>• May experience obsessions and compulsions at school. |
| 3. Identify his current motivators. | • Computer time.<br>• Praise for his work or just noticing and marveling at his accomplishments.<br>• Encouragement for his creative and inventive interests. |

**Key Aspects of a Behavior Plan for an AS Child with TS Tics (continued)**

| 4. Identify his best classroom | • If OC issues are present, implement strategies listed in Chapter Four.<br>• Provide a "refuge," "quiet area," or "reflection room," a space where the child may go when overwhelmed by the need to tic or perform a compulsion. This is a room at school that is comfortable, private, and possibly pre-stocked with some of the child's comfort items, such as a CD player, books, and writing materials or a computer.<br>• Allow the child to speak out. AS powered by the raw energy of TS gives a child an aggressive learning style. He benefits from having an actual conversation with his teacher and from verbal repartee in the class structured around the learning task.<br>• Allow the child to move around in the classroom or take movement breaks to use up some of the high-energy pressure he experiences, thereby enhancing his learning.<br>• Because of his tendency for OC, the child may be overly scrupulous and attempt to make every decision pertaining to him "perfectly fair." Help him deal with problems of social justice by talking about the "fairness" dilemmas you have encountered as a teacher.<br>• Build instruction around the child's interests, special or otherwise. The AS-plus-TS child has a difficult time marching to the drum of the instructional curriculum and learns best when he has to wrestle with a task or concept that he finds intrinsically interesting.<br>• Make sure teachers and substitutes know how to handle the AS-plus-TS child's tendency for moodiness, high anxiety, obsessionality, as well as the LDs that he may experience.<br>• Give the child lots of up-front time to prepare for changes in routine. Most AS-plus-TS children require a rigid daily routine. Allow extra time for completion of tasks, remove time limitations from tests, and provide a keyboard to complete writing assignments.<br>• Note overt or subtle provocations from other students. Quickly and quietly interrupt these activities. |
|---|---|

## Key Aspects of a Behavior Plan for an AS Child with TS Tics (continued)

| | |
|---|---|
| **5. Identify staff behaviors that are part of the solution – keeping the child focused and following.** | • Regular staff and substitute teachers are able to identify states of obsessionality, perfectionism, stress, and high anxiety. An obsessing child will seem out of focus and appear to look right through you. His eyes may track on the horizontal back and forth, indicating he is going over an obsessive introject in his mind. If a child becomes overly argumentative or rigid in his perceptions, he may be experiencing high anxiety. Once destabilized, he may become unmanageable for weeks or months. |
| | • Respect his privacy and pride. The best thing to do is to note the behavior that is problematic and privately ask the child if you can do something to help. This would be a time to implement positive aspects of a behavior plan, such as suggesting he go to his "refuge," go for a walk around the school, or run an errand. |
| | • Use empathetic language to bridge and redirect: "Nathan, you seem to be getting frustrated. How can I help?" Give him a choice that helps him deal with his frustration. |
| | • Redirect him if necessary. If agitation occurs because of a task requirement and he is not able to benefit from more explanation, ask him to complete a substitute activity. |
| **6. Identify staff behaviors that are part of the problem.** | • Do not show anger, embarrass him in front of the others, or demand compliance with a punishment threat. |
| | • Do not put task demands on the child when he is experiencing challenges related to his diagnosis. |
| | • Do not have inconsistent classroom rules, requirements, or unpredictability. |
| | • Do not ignore buildup in the child's frustration level due to misunderstanding of the task or directions. |
| | • Do not ignore taunting by other students. |

**Key Aspects of a Behavior Plan for an AS Child with TS Tics (continued)**

| 7. Identify action to be taken in the event his tics or OCs become intolerable. | • Use a matter-of-fact verbal style that normalizes the child's restlessness and does not put him down.<br><br>• Encourage use of the pass signal through which a child may notify his teacher that he needs to go to the reflection/refuge area to self-calm.<br><br>• Gently direct him to his refuge, where he can discharge tics and participate in other self-calming activity. If appropriate, let him take his desk work there and complete it there.<br><br>• Most children with the AS-plus-TS presentation do not require removal from school by parents to deal with issues. Tics and OC problems are medical conditions that should be addressed in the child's IEP in such a way that the child and his teacher can develop a plan to work on the reduction of their presence at school. Unlike the child with BD, the child with AS plus TS is not functionally disabled by overactivity of his brain's limbic system. Though it may take months and months of work and great patience, working with the child can produce the best positive outcome: He stays at school, keeps learning, and has friends among the other students and staff. |
|---|---|

## Conclusion: The Importance of Non-Isolating Emotional Support at School

Children with AS often feel a lack of control of their minds. They become disoriented in space and time and do not understand what others want from them. Children who experience motor and vocal tics and other "Touretticisms" are essentially out of control of their bodies. When both phenomena are present, the child may feel out of control of his mind *and* body, with nowhere to hide. If he were just challenged by AS, he could seek refuge in "nerdy" introversion at school, but the tics prevent him from having this option. Like it or not, his issues are evident to all and may be disturbing to many.

For this reason, caregivers of AS children who experience tics must be vigilant for the development of depression in the child and should take every opportunity to draw the child out of herself with supportive and helpful communication. In the same spirit, the child should not be expected to be in the spotlight at school unless she asks for this exposure.

It is important that a child not be isolated from her classmates because of her Tourette's-related challenges. It pains me to hear about children who are placed in self-contained classrooms with no other children present because of compulsive swearing and other disturbing motor or vocal tics. In these cases, a child's school decides that "administrative convenience" overrules the child's need for a good education in the least restrictive environment. I counsel parents to challenge such decisions and require schools to make accommodations for their children, to train staff in their management, and to educate other students about TS. Indeed, isolating a child may make his neurological and psychological issues more serious. Tourette's syndrome and its manifestations in AS children is an invitation to all caregivers to put aside their shocked reactions to a child's swearing or obscene vocalizations and to deal with the situation with the compassion and creativity the child deserves.

# Endnotes

139.  Sacks, O. (1985). *The man who mistook his wife for a hat.* New York: Summit Books. p. 233.
140.  Bruun, R. (1994). *A mind of its own.* New York: Oxford University Press. p. 155.
141.  Burd L., Fisher, W. W., Kerbeshian, J., & Arnold, M. E. (1987). Is the development of Tourette's Syndrome a marker for improvement in patients with autism and other developmental disorders? *Journal of the American Academy of Child and Adolescent Psychiatry, 26,* 162-165.
142.  Duran, M. (1998, November). *Tourette's syndrome and obsessive-compulsive behavior.* Annual conference of the Washington State Tourette's Syndrome Association, Seattle, WA.
143.  Sacks, O., with Siebert, E. (1995, May/June). A surgeon's life. *The Family Therapy Networker,* 62-63.
144.  Kruesi, M. (2005). Treatment of children with conduct disorder and aggression. In *What's new in child and adolescent psychiatry* (p. 74). Irving, CA: CME Inc.
145.  Berthier, M. L., Bayes, A., & Tolosa, E. S. (1993, May). Magnetic resonance imaging in patients with concurrent Tourette's Disorder and Asperger Syndrome. *Journal of the American Academy of Child and Adolescent Psychiatry, 32*(3), 633-639.
146.  Comings, D. (1991). *Tourette's syndrome and human behavior.* Duarte, CA: Hope Press. p. 626.
147.  Bruun, 1994.

148. Prigogine, I. (1977). *Self-organization in non-equilibrium systems: From dissipative structures to order through fluctuations.* New York: J. Wiley & Sons.
149. Cederlund & Gilberg, 2004.
150. Comings, D. (1991). p. 99; Freeman, R. D., Fast, D. K., Burd, L., Kerbeshian, J., Robertson, M. M., & Sandor P. (2000, July). An international perspective on Tourette's syndrome: Selected findings from 3,500 individuals in 22 countries. *Developmental Medicine & Child Neurology, 42,* 436-44.
151. Wilhelm, S., Deckersbach, T., Coffey, B. J., Bohne, A., Alan L. Peterson, A. L., & Lee Baer, L. (2003, June). Habit reversal versus supportive psychotherapy for Tourette's Disorder: A randomized controlled trial. *American Journal of Psychiatry, 160,* 1175-1177.
152. Vitiello, M. (1992). Doing it differently. In A. W. Seligman & J. S. Hilkevich, *Don't think about monkeys: Extraordinary stories by people with Tourette's.* Duarte, CA: Hope Press.
153. Lynn, 2000.

Chapter Eight

# So Close, So Far: Knowing the Difference Between ADD (Inattentive Type) and Asperger Syndrome

Quite a number of my young clients come in with a request from their teacher or school counselor to look at the possibility that the child has AS. Typically, school staff have noticed the child's isolation from other kids, poor self-organization, tendency toward angry hyperfocus, and brilliance in some specific area such as math, science, or art.

In my first session with the child I note that he looks Asperger-like. He has a difficult time expressing himself, tends to hyperfocus, seems anxious, and has sensory integration issues (SI). One telltale sign of his SI condition are the sweatpants he wears.

In my years of practice I have worked with many children like these, informally diagnosed as AS but really better fitting the ADD (inattentive type) diagnosis. I understand the confusion. All the noted features make the child look as if AS challenges him. But I have learned to respect the statistic: ADD is five times more prevalent than AS, and although a child looks as if he has AS, there is a much better chance that ADD is the issue. A word about this diagnosis is in order.

Inattentive ADD is defined with the same symptoms as ADHD in the DSM IV (314.01) except for the absence of hyperactivity. In my clinical experience, the child challenged by ADD Inattentive Type also experiences hyperactivity, although it is his mind, not his body, that is hyperactive. Many persons with ADD Inattentive Type note that, although they appear calm on the outside, there is a "cyclone" going on inside. The day-to-day challenges that the ADD child faces include distractibility, inattention, problems doing things that are not interesting to them (activation), memory problems, and hyperactivity.

Children with AS face all the "executive function" challenges of children with ADD. They tend to be inattentive, distractible, moody, and to have poor short-term memory. They also have a very difficult time with brain activation at times of transition – they hate to change their routines and need a lot of up-front warning that something is about to happen.

While the day-to-day challenges of the child with AS may include executive function problems, he faces additional challenges, such as social isolation, loneliness, and an almost total lack of common sense. It is important to decide the AS or ADD question early in the child's life because children of each neurotype need different types of support at home and at school. Here are five important dimensions of their characterological difference.

## Four Essential Differences Between Asperger Syndrome and Attention Deficit Disorder

1. **The emotional lives of the child with AS and the child with ADD are markedly different.**

   A defining feature of AS is a difference in the way the child experiences and expresses emotion. ADD children have neurotypical emotional lives, children with AS do not. This marked difference makes exploration of the child's emotional being the first order of business.

   The child challenged by ADD is emotionally delayed. The 15-year-old child with ADD may have the emotional age of an 11-year-old but, given this delay, he has a full range of social and emotional capability. The child challenged by AS speaks the language of logic, not emotion, and is therefore less equipped for getting his emotional needs met.

   I use the word "illiterate" to refer to the emotional functioning of children with AS to denote the fact that the child cannot read the emotional language of others and also has a very difficult time understanding his own emotional states. He is able to express "I am angry," "I am very frustrated,"

"I am frightened," and, sometimes, "I am sad," but he typically does not express more complex emotional states. For example, if you asked him after he had a verbal exchange with his mom, "How did that feel to you? Did her words hurt you when she said you were a mean boy?," he would not be able to tell you. Though a younger child, AS or ADD, would probably not be able to answer this question either, most ADD adolescents would say, "Yes. It hurt when she said that. She has never said that I was a mean person before." To learn a language you have to be able to compare meanings of words, building bridges from the familiar to the unfamiliar. The child with AS is severely impaired in his ability to assign words to his own emotional meanings and cross-compare them with others.

The child with AS will show a poor understanding of what motivates other children and adults in his life, whereas the child with ADD may have an excellent understanding of the motivations of others. It is not his lack of understanding, but his impulsivity and inattention, that gets him in trouble with other people.

The child who inhabits the AS neurotype is not moved by emotion; he is moved by thoughts, or by visions perhaps. The word "emotion" broken into its two essential parts "e" and "motion" describes the impact of feeling on action. We do what we feel moved to do. For many children with AS, life is about doing your work, not about feeling good.

The ADD child more than likely has a low "emotional IQ" – his chronological age is higher than his emotional age. A good rule of thumb is that emotional age equals two thirds of chronological age. That is, if the child is 15 years old, his emotional age is 10 or 11. His emotional underdevelopment shows in his social impulsivity, irritability, and inability to keep friends. However, he has a rich emotional life aside from these issues. He may be very empathetic, and he is capable of give-and-take in conversation and repairing conversation when embarrassments occur or blurts happen. It may not be easy for him, but he is capable of doing it if he has to.

When I am having the kind of strategic conversation with a child that leads to accurate diagnosis, I am conscious of the quality of his emotional contact with me. I am not primarily concerned with eye contact. If a child makes no direct eye contact with me, I note the fact. Nevertheless, I do not consider lack of eye contact diagnostic of AS because I have met as many AS kids who have good eye contact as do not. If the child is capable of bantering with me, or joking around or teasing me, I put a check mark in the "probable ADD" column. This kind of conversational volleying is very difficult for children challenged by AS.

In terms of brain function, research indicates that there are differences in the way that people with AS and people with ADD process emotional information. People with ADD as a stand-alone issue show abnormality of function in the frontal lobes of the brain but no abnormality in the way that their limbic systems process emotional events such as the recognition of emotional states in another's face. People with AS and HFA show abnormalities in this task – they tend to assign the same importance to the recognition of an inanimate object such as a car as to the recognition of a person's face, and their brains do not activate if that face shows strong emotion such as terror, fear, or happiness.[154]

If a child makes no eye contact, I may ask him what he experiences when he looks away from someone. If he tells me, "I cannot think and make eye contact at the same time," I will consider the possibility that the child's AS-related tendency for "fixed-figure" perception is interfering with his ability to do two things at one time – making eye contact and thinking.

I learn a lot about a child by asking him about his friends. If all his friends are "nerds" or "computer geeks," I put a check in the "look further for AS" box. Typically, AS kids enjoy productive fun together centered on an activity. For them, there is not as much give-and-take and interpersonal banter as exists between children who inhabit the ADD pattern. Go to any large shopping mall where the kids hang out, and you will see the neurotypicals and ADD kids doing the same thing – teasing each other, flirting, and bragging. You will not typically see a child with AS doing these things.

The child with AS is more likely to experience meltdown. This total loss of composure and disintegration of coping ability occurs when she is painfully frustrated. By comparison, the child with ADD is more typically given to a chronic irritability that can often be focused as angry outbursts. However, through it all, the child will be in control of his reaction.

The child with ADD may tend to become fixated on things or to hyperfocus on them, but he does not have obsessions. By contrast, many children with AS experience obsessions and compulsions. Definitional of an obsession is the fact that it pushes a person to perform a compulsion out of dread of an unknown penalty. The person has the sense that if he does not obey the obsessional demand, he, or others, will be severely harmed. The hyper-focused child with ADD becomes visually entranced or cognitively stuck on an activity such as playing a video game (the most typical example given to me by parents), but his fixation is not driven by a sense of dread. Brain scans of children with ADD who hyperfocus show that there is over-activity in the cingulate cortex of the brain.[155] This structure has a role in driving perseverance, the repetition of thought, feeling, and action seen in OCD and TS. But, unlike the child with OCD, the child with ADD does not experience the cognitive ingredient (the feeling-thought "If I do not obey, something dreadful will happen.").

All children with AS may not experience obsessions and compulsions, but they are much more likely to do so than kids with ADD. In Chapter Four, I described the difference between the special interests and obses-sional states of children with AS. The most dramatic difference to note here is that compulsions are pushed by the obsessional demand to "even things up." The child experiences the felt need to "make something right" that is not. A special interest is pushed by the child's fascination with some subject and desire to learn everything there is to know about it. The AS child will appear obsessed with her special interest but is able to control her enthusi-asm (she can if he must). The obsessing child does not have this choice – it is truly "do it or die" to him.

2. **In terms of approach to tasks, children with AS tend to be special-ists, whereas children with ADD tend to be generalists.**
I define a child's cognitive style as the way she typically solves prob-lems. The child challenged by ADD and the child challenged by AS demonstrate two essential differences in their problem-solving ap-proaches.

The child with AS shows great strength in recognizing the details of function of one particular technology or has deep knowledge of one particular subject area. She will enjoy analysis of known facts in her special interest and cross-association of these facts. She will have a difficult time generalizing to other domains of inquiry or effort. As suggested elsewhere in this book, she is the one who you want to be "defusing the bomb," the one to count on when it is important to make those tiny discriminations of detail. She has significant strength in noticing details about something and significant talent as a "logical detective." The child challenged by ADD, on the other hand, will more likely use an intuitive, feelings-based, approach to problem solving. And, he will take other people into consideration when solving a problem or making a decision.

The AS child, given the task of solving some problem in his science class, will define the problem with precision and sort through all possible solutions in sequence to get to the correct answer. Being a powerful visual thinker, he will do these calculations mentally and will not write out the steps to the solution in any detail. By comparison, the ADD child would be more likely to free-associate possibilities and experiment creatively with different combinations until he gets a solution that "feels right." If he were working on a team with other kids, he would pay attention to their solutions and either accept them or banter with them to get his point across. Many AS children would continue to argue, insisting they are correct, not being able to let go of the issue until others have conceded that they were wrong.

With regard to perceptual style, the child with ADD shows an ability to range wide and far on the topic and free-associate different aspects of the problem around a central question. As I have noted before, the child with AS uses a fixed-figure perceptual style and has a lot of difficulty generalizing to other topics. He is the ultimate specialist and may be a good balance to the free-form creativity of the ADD child.

3.  **Children with AS tend to have one special interest, whereas children with ADD have ever-changing interests.**
    A child with AS seeks to know all that there is to know about a special interest. This interest may last throughout his childhood and into young adulthood or it may diminish and something else may come to the fore to inspire his passion. The strength of the AS child lies in his cognitive resolve, his ability to go deep into analysis of something to see its interconnected parts.

    The ADD child will not show presence of a special interest and will not have the ability to go as deep into the topic. He will go wide, not deep, relating to the world as an artist with many projects going in his studio at the same time.

4. **The essential talents and delights of the child with AS are different from those of the child with ADD.**

Unlike the ADD child who may experience delight in some physical activity such as skate boarding, dance, or some artistic activity, the child with AS delights in making something work better. He is typically fascinated with lists and specifications. He loves games like *Trivial Pursuit* and the recitation of "useless facts." He will be a force to be reckoned with should he choose to play on a TV game show. By comparison, the child with ADD will not voice this delight in mastering categories, and he will be quickly bored with *Trivial Pursuit*-types of games, and with the acquisition of information.

The following table summarizes the major differences between children with AS and those with ADD.

**Asperger Syndrome and Attention Deficit Disorder
(Inattentive Type): Markers of Difference**

| Domain | AS/PDD | ADD |
|---|---|---|
| **1. The social and emotional lives of the child with AS and the child with ADD are markedly different.** | • Emotionally "illiterate." Impaired ability to understand the emotional life of others or label own emotional states.<br><br>• Highly logical; thoughts before feelings.<br><br>• OC behavior common.<br><br>• Meltdown much more common.<br><br>• Assigns same meaning to human faces as to objects.<br><br>• Cannot "be social" and "think" at the same time.<br><br>• Cannot engage in banter and give-and-take in conversation. | • Emotional immaturity contributes to short friendships.<br><br>• Highly emotional; feelings before thoughts – the "Ready, fire, aim" approach.<br><br>• OC behaviors not as common.<br><br>• Chronic irritability.<br><br>• Negative thought fixation but is not obsessive-compulsive.<br><br>• Capable of give-and-take in conversation and repairing conversation after blurting.<br><br>• May be socially impulsive and overly aggressive. |

## Asperger Syndrome and Attention Deficit Disorder
## (Inattentive Type): Markers of Difference (continued)

| Domain | AS/PDD | ADD |
|---|---|---|
| **2. The AS child is a specialist. The ADD child is a generalist.** | • Shows evidence of having a fixed-figure, parts-only (not parts-to-whole) perceptual style.<br><br>• Has an exceptional recall for details and notices things others do not.<br><br>• The ultimate specialist. | • Impulsivity, distractibility, inattention, memory, activation.<br><br>• Mental hyperactivity.<br><br>• Whole-to-parts perceptual style.<br><br>• Solves problems by playing with information, to see relationships and creative connections. |
| **3. The AS child has a special interest. The ADD child has ever-changing interests.** | • Strong persistent interests.<br><br>• Cannot address other topics. | • Ever-changing interests. |
| **4. The essential talents and delights of the child with AS and the child with ADD are different.** | • Fascinated with lists and specifications.<br><br>• Delights in new learning about special interest, "useless facts," and mind trivia.<br><br>• Delights in flawless function.<br><br>• Difficulty dealing with novelty. | • Delights in new experiences, athletics and the performing and visual arts. |

## Conclusion: Get to Know a Child to See Clear Differences Between the ADD and AS Neurotypes

Children with ADD may be assumed to have "Asperger's" for a variety of reasons. They may be highly anxious and demonstrate the tendency toward oppositionality or phobic behavior often seen in children with the AS diagnosis. Some ADD children get fixated on things to the point of being unable to stop what they are doing. This may look like the will and focus the AS child brings to his special interest. Further, many children with ADD are highly oppositional and combative. This may cause the child to be socially isolated and similar to the child with AS in this regard.

In order to understand the child and her issues and appropriate diagnosis, you must spend time with her and get to know her joys and sorrows. All too often diagnosis is made by one professional based on a read of the results of some other professional, and very little actual time is spent in the presence of the child. In my experience, this mistake is made often in considering whether a child is properly diagnosed as ADD or AS.

Spending time with a child enables you to look past her symptoms to know what is really going on with her. Perhaps she has been diagnosed with AS because she does not make eye contact or carry the conversation at all. However, suddenly you notice that when she is relaxed, she is very interactional and socially effective. She just has a mild social phobia that makes for a world-class wallflower.

Or perhaps he has been diagnosed with ADD because he does not show the pronounced social stress, withdrawal, or learning problems typical of children with AS. He "has a couple of friends." Then you notice that for all the months you have known him, he has talked of nothing but his collection of little army men, one video game, or his interest in computers. As you delve into his life at school, you realize that his social success there is more a result of his proficiency in some activity the other kids value (such as maintaining the school's computer network) than it is of any social ability. In fact, he is unable to initiate conversation or banter with other kids and his two "best friends" are science buddies at school whom he never sees outside that setting. Here we have an AS child who has used his considerable intelligence to "pass" for neurotypical. It can be done. Many of the children we discuss in this book have powerful intelligences, and this is a huge plus when it comes to figuring out how to compensate for neurological challenges.

The behavioral differences between these two types are subtle. As parents and professionals, we are best advised to go slow and to invite the child to tell us her own story so that we can see who she is and how we can best help her. When I have erred in my own evaluations of kids in this regard, it has been because of impatience. Children are not their diagnoses; they are complete personalities. I have learned that it is sometimes best to drop my initial focus on diagnostic patterns and just get to know a child. Once I have established rapport, which may take many sessions of counseling, aspects of an appropriate diagnosis will simply present themselves.

## Endnotes

154. Critchley, H. D. et al. (2002, November). The functional neuroanatomy of social behavior: changes in cerebral blood flow when people with autistic disorder process facial expressions. *Brain*, 2203-2212.

155. Amen, 2001.

## Chapter Nine

# Using the Character Map to Identify a Child's Neurotype

I n this chapter, I provide a decision tree, a set of "go, no-go" prompts to guide you to the appropriate diagnosis for a child. This assessment uses short "yes" or "no" question sets for each of the neurotypes discussed in this book. You can begin your own inquiry by going through the features often seen in AS and then branch out from there to see if features of other neurotypes are present. These features are listed in the questionnaire called the Character Map.

The Character Map contains diagnostic criteria (symptoms listed in the DSM-IV) and "soft" criteria – identifying characteristics of children diagnosed with AS and associated conditions that are not listed in the DSM-IV but are found often in testing and clinical practice. It does not list every symptom for each diagnosis. The Character Map is not a primary guide for DSM-IV diagnosis. It is intended to illustrate the patterns of character and neurological type of children with difficult behavior and to provide creative inspiration for diagnostic assessment.

The Character Map first surveys features seen in AS as a stand-alone condition. Then it lists traits of personality seen in children who evidence an AS-plus neurotype – BD, NLD, OCD, and ODD. Finally, it compares and contrasts AS with three look-alike conditions – HFA, ADD, and TS.

Scoring is not complicated. In Part I, score the child for presence of the "must have" characteristics of AS. Then look over the shaded features listed for each of the first four AS-plus diagnostic categories (BD, NLD, OCD, and ODD). Given that the child's life shows presence of the shaded factors identified for AS, note any of the Asperger-plus categories that accurately describe him.

Part II contains descriptions of neurotypes that look like AS but are not AS and cannot logically co-exist with AS. Use this part if you want to evaluate the child for the presence of AS *or* HFA, ADD, or TS.

For the purpose of this book and the Character Map, AS is not considered "a mild form of autism." AS and autism look a lot alike but children with each of these conditions have markedly different perceptual styles (see distinctions listed in Chapter Six). Likewise, a child cannot be diagnosed with both AS and ADD. This is a logical impossibility. The attentional deficits seen in AS are profound and much more severe than those seen in ADD. The brain structures involved are different (ADD is related to issues with brain frontal lobe function, AS involves the frontal lobes and structures in the limbic system such as the hippocampus and amygdala). With regard to TS, children with AS may show the two central symptoms of TS – motor and vocal tics – *and* have all the other AS-related symptoms. The only valid diagnosis is TS as a stand-alone issue or AS with tics.

Once a diagnostic pattern is identified, consult the relevant chapter in the book to review strategies for helping a child who fits the particular neurotype.

## Essential Features of Asperger Syndrome

Here is the basic template we use to compare and contrast AS with other diagnostic categories. Check "yes" or "no" to evaluate presence of each factor. Shaded factors must be present to fit the AS neurotype.

You will note that neurotypes may share some features (e.g., in both AS and HFA there are social skills impairments). And there will be features that are only listed for a particular neurotype. These are key features – aspects of a child's experience and behavior that I weigh heavily when considering the fit for a particular diagnosis. These key features are shaded in the questionnaires.

## Essential Features of Asperger Syndrome

| | Yes | No |
|---|---|---|
| **I. Impairment in social interaction as indicated by at least two of the following:** | | |
| Impairment in the use of nonverbal behaviors such as eye contact, facial expression, body postures, and gestures. | | |
| Failure to develop peer relationships. | | |
| Lack of spontaneous seeking to share enjoyments and interests. | | |
| Lack of social or emotional reciprocity. | | |
| **II. Restricted pattern of behavior as indicated by at least of the following:** | | |
| Presence of a special interest that is abnormal in intensity and focus. | | |
| Inflexible adherence to nonfunctional routines or rituals. | | |
| Stereotypical and repetitive motor mannerisms (hand flapping, finger twisting). | | |
| Preoccupation with parts of objects. | | |
| **III. No clinically significant delays in language, cognitive development, self-help skills, and interest in the environment.** | | |
| **Other features drawn from the author's obvservations of his clients with the diagnosis (not from the DSM IV):** | | |
| At least one immediate relative also shows presence of the features noted above. | | |
| Is interested primarily in things and ideas and the relationships between objects not between people. | | |
| Tends to be cognitively rigid and inflexible – a black-and-white thinker. | | |
| Perceptual style is "fixed figure." When approaching an interesting object, he is impaired in the ability see the context or background around the object – his focus is fixed only on that object and he does not move easily between it and other objects in the field. He cannot see "the forest through the trees" and will get stuck on One Special Tree that will become his "fixation." | | |
| **Characteristic gifts:** He makes systems work better. He is the ultimate technologist. | | |

## Part I: Asperger-Plus Clusters

Clusters 1-4 list characteristic features of conditions that often co-occur with AS. Evaluate the child for the possibility of the AS-plus diagnosis by checking "yes" or "no" to the descriptors for the child in each cluster. A child with a primary diagnosis of AS may show features of one or more of these companion conditions.

## Cluster 1: Distinguishing Characteristics of Children with AS plus BD

| Domain | Yes | No |
|---|---|---|
| **Meets diagnostic criteria for AS and ...** | | |
| Shows presence of:<br><br>a. Mood swing from mania or hypomania to a state of clinical depression. And/or<br><br>b. is seen as a "mixed state" in which both moods are present at the same time (often noted as chronic serious irritability that devolves into rage). | | |
| **Other features noted in the clinical setting:** | | |
| Has at least one immediate relative clearly diagnosed with BD. | | |
| Shows presence of psychosis and/or disordered thought process. | | |
| Is very distractible and inattentive. | | |
| Special interest may express psychosis or hypomania such as computer system cracking, mixing dangerous chemicals, and other dangerous activities. | | |
| Is chronically irritable and hyper-reactive to criticism. | | |
| Has few good friends. | | |
| Refuses to go to school. | | |
| Tends to take dangerous risks. | | |
| Has obsessions and compulsions. | | |
| Becomes hypomanic in the evening. | | |
| Goes out at night to enjoy colors, cooler temperature, and absence of others. | | |
| May have a tendency for angry asexuality and hyper-morality or have difficulty with sexual impulsivity. | | |
| Is verbally aggressive. | | |
| Shows presence of sensory integration problems. | | |
| Voices suicidal thoughts. | | |
| **Characteristic gifts:**<br>• Able to apply powerful and focused energy toward the accomplishment of goals.<br><br>• Unusual creativity in technical and artistic endeavors. | | |

*Note.* Shaded factors *must* be present to fit the BD neurotype.

## Cluster 2: Distinguishing Characteristics of AS Plus NLD

| Domain | Yes | No |
|---|---|---|
| **Meets diagnostic criteria for AS and ...** | | |
| Is unable to process nonverbal information. He must hear it to remember it. | | |
| **Other features noted in the clinical setting:** | | |
| Has an excellent auditory rote memory. | | |
| Has a low tolerance for novelty and change. | | |
| Is physically uncoordinated. As a young child, could not tie shoes. | | |
| Cannot solve open-ended problems creatively. Works best with known variables. | | |
| Low proficiency in science and math unless problems are presented verbally. | | |
| Prefers sedentary work to physically demanding work. | | |
| In educational settings, has severe content retention problems and requires daily review of material covered previously. | | |
| **Characteristic gifts:**<br>• Excels in debate and singing.<br><br>• May be excellent speller and possess advanced vocabulary skills.<br><br>• Is very good at solving problems with known variables such as logic problems.<br><br>• Is the ultimate archivist; very strong skills in librarianship. | | |

*Note.* Shaded factors *must* be present to fit the NLD neurotype.

## Cluster 3: Distinguishing Characteristics of Children with AS Plus OCD

| Domain | Yes | No |
|---|---|---|
| **Meets diagnostic criteria for AS and ...** | | |
| Experiences obsessive thought or the need to do certain things and compulsions – behaviors enacted to avoid some danger or sense of dread. | | |
| **Other features noted in the clinical setting:** | | |
| Has a strong tendency to get locked into negative thoughts or is unable to dissociate from the memory of some negative event. | | |
| Appears severely distracted and inattentive, staring into space. This inattention is not a result of ADD or other clinical conditions that produce extreme distractibility (such as BD). | | |
| Becomes extremely upset, to the point of meltdown, when asked to pay attention. | | |
| Complains of not being able to sleep at night because of recurring "stupid thoughts" that he cannot get out of his mind. | | |
| Is generally harm-avoidant and anxious. Refuses to go to school from time to time. Is afraid to be alone in the house. | | |
| **Characteristic gifts:**<br>• Great perseverance in the pursuit of personal goals.<br><br>• Extremely careful with the details of a project; does not miss the important fine points. The ideal "scientific" personality.<br><br>• Scrupulous, honest, and protective of others. | | |

*Note.* Shaded factors *must* be present to fit the OCD neurotype.

## Cluster 4: Distinguishing Characteristics of Children with AS Plus ODD

| Domain | Yes | No |
|---|---|---|
| **Meets diagnostic criteria for AS and ...** | | |
| Most always refuses caregivers' requests. Is combative, chronically angry, touchy, and easily annoyed by others. | | |
| **Other features noted in the clinical setting:** | | |
| Has low frustration tolerance, loses temper frequently and easily. | | |
| Reports unspecified anxiety, fear of humiliation, or separation anxiety. | | |
| Is subject to uncontrollable worry. | | |
| Has a fear for own safety and difficulty concentrating as a result. | | |
| Complains of muscle tension, stomachache, and headache. Fatigues easily. | | |
| Shows presence of sensory integration problems. | | |
| **Characteristic gifts:**<br>• Capacity for great resolve, emotional strength, and loyalty to friends. May be very troublesome to adversaries. | | |

*Note.* Shaded factors *must* be present to fit the ODD neurotype.

### Scoring

Review the "yes" and "no" responses you gave to the traits described for each neurotype. Identify the probable core neurotype as the one in which you could check "yes" for the core shaded features. Assign 1 point for each associated factor (unshaded items) in the diagnosis checked "yes."

1. How many points did you assign to each neurotype? _____

2. Which is the more probable neurotype? _____

# Part II: Differentiating "Look-Alike" Conditions: Asperger Syndrome *or* High-Functioning Autism

Typically, children with HFA show presence of the DSM-IV symptoms listed under I or II below. In addition, the HFA child shows presence of the features noted as III below. It is the presence of these additional symptoms that suggests the more profound diagnosis of HFA is appropriate.

## Cluster 5: Core Features of High-Functioning Autism in Children

| I. Qualitative impairment in social interaction as shown by the presence of at least two of the following: | Yes | No |
|---|---|---|
| Impairment in the use of nonverbal behaviors such as eye contact, facial expression, body postures, and gestures. | | |
| Failure to develop peer relationships. | | |
| Lack of spontaneous seeking to share enjoyments and interests. | | |
| Lack of social or emotional reciprocity. | | |
| II. Qualitative impairment in communication as shown by the presence of at least one of the following (*before age 3): | | |
| *Delay in the development of spoken language. | | |
| *If language is present, marked impairment in the ability to initiate and sustain a conversation. | | |
| Stereotypical and repetitive use of language. | | |
| * Lack of make-believe or socially imitative play. | | |
| III. Restricted pattern of behavior as shown by the presence of at least one of the following: | | |
| Presence of a special interest that is abnormal in intensity and focus. | | |
| Inflexible adherence to nonfunctional routines or rituals. | | |
| Stereotypical and repetitive motor mannerisms (hand flapping, finger twisting). | | |
| Persistent preoccupation with parts of objects. | | |

## Cluster 5: Core Features of High-Functioning Autism in Children (continued)

| IV. Other features (often, not always) noted in a clinical setting (from birth to age 6): | Yes | No |
|---|---|---|
| Does not follow finger point when adult says, "look there!" | | |
| Does not make eye contact or verbally interact with parents. | | |
| Appears to be happily self-contained and not interested in other people. | | |
| In some cases, the child seemed to be developing normally and then, suddenly began enacting behaviors  noted here. | | |
| **Other features noted in the clinical setting (age 7 to 18):** | | |
| Is visual thinker. Does not think in words to represent information and solve problems. | | |
| Demonstrates a need to separate himself from others to achieve a sense of stimulus safety. | | |
| **Other features drawn from the author's observations of his clients with the diagnosis (not from the DSM-IV or other research):** | | |
| The child's perceptual style shows evidence of "full-field" perceptual style. He takes things around him in as complete "wholes." He sees only the forest and not the trees, and he is perceptually overwhelmed by the rush of stimuli coming at him. He has great difficulty separating individual objects of focus from their background. | | |
| **Characteristic gifts:**<br>• Visionary, mystic, or breakthrough thinker in the arts and sciences.<br>• Savantic skills in math and science.<br>• Savantic visual-kinesthetic memory; may remember exact details from one day years in the past.<br>• Savantic skills as visual artist; able to exactly replicate subject of study. | | |

## How Is the Child with AS Essentially Different from the Child with HFA?

- The child with AS has a "fixed-figure" perceptual style, the child with HFA has a "full-field" perceptual style.

- He is able to think in both words and pictures. The child with HFA is an exclusive visual thinker.

- He has some capability for word-based imagination and creativity.

- He can accurately track the passage of time (the clock is a device that uses language to communicate its meaning). The child with HFA will seem lost in space and time.

- He can use language to express inner states, feelings, and beliefs.

- He can *think* logically and analytically using language to represent information.

### Examples

- The AS child will perseverantly discuss his special interest in class. The child with HFA will seem to "space out" and rarely contribute to the discussion.

- At school, the AS child will be bossy and hypersensitive to any criticism of his bossiness. The HFA child will avoid conflict of any kind and seem to be in a world of his own.

- The HFA child will show extreme aversions to stimulation at school, such as background noise, smells, and crowding. The child with AS may complain about these issues but will be able to function O.K., though distracted and irritable.

## Cluster 6: Asperger Syndrome or Tourette's Syndrome

### Core Features of Tourette's Syndrome in Children

| Domain | Yes | No |
|---|---|---|
| a. Has verbal and motor tics that have been present for over a year. | | |
| b. Does not meet diagnostic criteria for any other disorder. | | |
| **Other features noted in a clinical setting:** | | |
| Shows low "emotional IQ" – has difficulty reading others' emotional states. | | |
| Has poor distance boundaries; gets too close to other children. | | |
| Has obsessions and compulsions. | | |
| Enjoys wrestling, body contact sports, and sculpture. | | |
| Shows features of AD/HD or ADD. | | |
| Repeats words, actions of others. | | |
| Engages in coprolalia (compulsive repetition of obscenities). | | |
| In elementary school-aged children, enjoys scatological humor (more than the average child does). | | |
| **Characteristic gifts:**<br>• Creative thought; unusual solutions; loves to ask "what if?" types of questions.<br><br>• Musical invention. Drum players.<br><br>• Connected with all things natural and earthy.<br><br>• Physically quick. | | |

## How Is the Child with AS Different from the Child with TS?

- The child with AS has a highly logical communication style. The child with TS tends to be highly emotional.

- The child with AS may show profound communication deficits. The child with TS will more likely show neurotypical ability to understand the intentions of others and react appropriately.

- The child with AS is good at technical and scientific invention. The child with TS favors artistic invention.

- The child with AS may be poorly coordinated and is not physically fast. Children with TS are often gifted with athletic agility and speed.

### Examples

- The AS child will be drawn to the Computer Club or Chess Club. The child with TS will be drawn to wrestling, track, or soccer.

- The child with AS will speak in an expressionless monotone. The child with TS will appear animated, engaged, and enjoy argument.

## Cluster 7: AS or ADD (Inattentive Type)

| Domain | Yes | No |
|---|---|---|
| **The ADD child (this is a clinical definition, not the DSM-IV diagnosis)** | | |
| Possesses "executive function" deficits. A. Poor short-term memory, B. Distractibility, C. Inattention, D. Brain activation problems (see first feature listed below), E. Chronic moodiness and hypersensitivity | | |
| **Other features noted in a clinical setting:** | | |
| Is highly emotional – feelings before thoughts. | | |
| Has a tendency toward negative thought fixation. | | |
| Is emotionally immature. | | |
| Is personally disorganized. | | |
| Has poor impulse control. | | |
| Has shifting (not "special") interests. | | |
| Is highly creative. | | |
| Mental or physical hyperactivity – reports sense of "inner storm" or "brain noise." | | |
| **Characteristic gifts:** Creativity in art, music, and design. AD/HD children tend to be creative managers and leaders. | | |

*Note.* Shaded factors *must* be present to fit the ADD neurotype.

### How Is the Child with AS Essentially Different from the Child with ADD?

- He is or emotionally *illiterate.* The ADD child is emotionally *delayed.*

- *Thoughts* move the AS child to action. *Feelings* move the ADD child to action.

- The AS child often experiences obsessions and compulsions, the ADD child rarely experiences obsessions and compulsions.

- The AS child has a significant strength in the noticing of details about something and significant talent as a "logical detective." The ADD child may be distractible and inattentive to details.

- The AS child tends to be formalistic and rigid. The ADD child tends to be spontaneous and uninhibited.

- The AS child talks down to listeners as if he is a professor and they are his students. The ADD child may be loquacious and verbally unorganized.

- The AS child has one special interest to which he will devote all his spare time. The child with ADD has interests that shift, and he may not complete projects.

- The AS child delights in the acquisition of information. The ADD child delights in physical adventure – doing things he has never done before.

## Examples

- The frustrated ADD child may "flip off" his teacher and stalk off angrily. The frustrated AS student may have a major meltdown, throwing over his desk and threatening others.

- When divided into task teams, the ADD child may serve as leader, harmonizer, or bringer of humor. The AS child will serve the role of information provider and quality control specialist.

- The speech of the ADD child may ramble and he may be too loquacious. The AS child will stay on topic, will lack emotional expression, and go on too long. The ADD child may reflexively check in with his listener to see if he is getting across. The AS child will rarely do this kind of cross-check and will assume listeners understand his meaning.

## Scoring

Identify the probable core neurotype as the one in which you could check "yes" for all items that are shaded (required features for diagnosis). Then add up the total points of the unshaded items, assigning 1 point for each question.

Which is the more probable neurotype? _____

## Character Mapping Seeks the Child's "Distinctive Mark"

The desired result from completing the Character Map is greater understanding of the child's "character." This term and the term "diagnosis" are not synonymous. "Diagnosis" is a medical term used to denote how a person is sick. The word "character" is derived from the Greek to mean, "A distinctive mark impressed on something." The child's genius, his individual spirit, makes the distinctive mark that we seek with this process. Using the Character Map, we seek to identify both the challenges and gifts so that we may learn how to build the power of the child's gifts within his life.

Conclusion

# Seeing the Spirit of a Child Through His Diagnosis

Caregivers show disrespect for a child if they attempt to identify the child's diagnosis or genius solely by completing a battery of tests or an interview in a psychologist's office. The word "respect" is drawn from the Latin word "respicare," which means "to look at again." In order to know any child, you must look at her many times from your heart and your head and resist the urge to foreclose on a conclusion that may be based on preconception.

Diagnostic criteria are the tip of the iceberg. Getting an accurate idea of a particular child's neurotype is only the first step to understanding who he is, but it is an important first step.

It is important that we adults in our roles as parents, teachers, therapists, and other caregivers fight our tendency to pigeonhole a child by his symptoms. The truth is we really don't know what he is experiencing on the inside. The truth is also that if we listen with patience and a certain detached love, we may become enriched by our intuitive emotional knowing of the child. In this state of consciousness, in warm dialogue and reflection that occurs over time, we begin not only to see the outlines of the child's appropriate diagnosis, but are able to go beneath this medical term to see his gifts and true character.

Given this warning against reducing a child's personality to a machine that can be observed and adjusted to function better, there are good reasons for understanding his specific neurotype, the patterns of thought, feeling, and action that come into being as a result of his brain development. The better we know his pattern of gifts and challenges, the better we are able to parent him, offer educational services, provide appropriate medication, and enlist other support services such as counseling to get him through to adulthood, at which time he may decide on his own what kind of pharmacology best serves him.

Every child is different in this regard. No one method for parenting is right for every child. No one author or therapist has all the answers. It is very important to custom-tailor our approach to every child so as not to undervalue his ability to comply or to overwhelm him with unrealistic expectations.

We hope that this book is useful to parents, teachers, and other caregivers in their attempts to accurately classify patterns or personality of children with AS and other diagnoses. Once this is done, we move to the point of helping the child, and this involves getting a clearer idea of his gifts. This is why we have put so much emphasis in this book on the positive features of children with AS, BD, NLD, OCD, ODD, HFA, TS, ADD, and other neurotypes. Although we acknowledge the challenges these children face, no one ever improved himself or herself just by looking at what is "wrong." We all need a positive vision so that we can give a child more of what makes his life successful and keeps his focus on that success pattern.

Dr. James Hillman, a Jungian psychiatrist, studied the character peculiarities of people he called the "most eminent personalities of the 20th century." Hillman[156] suggests that *all* were neurologically different, odd, wild, and noncomforming. Many showed features of Asperger Syndrome and other conditions described in this book.

Looking back on Hillman's list, we see that the master healers, inventors, artists, and writers of the last 100 years were all people who had "severe behavior issues" when they were children and most hated school. As we have noted before, these eminent personalities were not necessarily "nice" people or "happy" people, for that matter. However, if you looked at them with soft and loving eyes, you could see their *genius* from a very young age.

People like Thomas Edison, Nikola Tesla, Howard Hughes, and Georgia O'Keeffe wanted "real tools" as children (to quote Nobel Laureate Dr. Barbara McClintock, a likely candidate for AS). They wanted to get on with it; to do what they came to do with their lives. Many of them weren't much fun to be around but their energy was interesting and avid for accomplishment.

The job of parenting our kids often feels thankless. This is regrettable because if the world could do so, it would thank these caregivers for cultivating the ones who bring *disturbance* to our planet. The systems theorist Ilya Prigogine[157] taught us that systems that become static, that do not change, die. Systems that stay healthy do so as a result of a balance between stability and disturbance. Our children, when all is said and done, are like the hurricanes that – when the devastation is over – refresh and renew the land. These children look at everything with fresh vision and do not accept conventional answers. They fight absurdity and will not tolerate it even if they find this absurdity in a school system that professes to teach "free-thinking" but is itself abhorrent of the practice.

The intention of this book is to support parents and other caregivers to provide a clearer vision of the talents, genius, and challenges of children with AS and its co-occurring conditions so that as disturbing as our kids' behavior can be, we are able to avoid pathologizing them so as to see past their symptoms. In so doing, we awaken the brilliance in them, the mind light that eventually becomes strong enough for them to find their own way in the world.

## Endnotes

156. Hillman, J. (1996). *The soul's code: In search of character and calling.* New York: Random House.
155. Prigogine, 1997.

# References

Abramowitz, J. S., Whiteside, S. P., & Deacon, B. J. (2005). The effectiveness of treatment for pediatric obsessive-compulsive disorder. A meta-analysis. *Behavior Therapy, 36*, 55-63.

Akiskal, H. S. (1995, June). Developmental pathways to bipolarity: Are juvenile-onset depressions pre-bipolar? *Journal of the American Academy of Child and Adolescent Psychiatry, 34*(6), 754-763.

Amen, D. (2001). *Healing ADD*. New York: Berkley Books.

American Psychiatric Association. (2000). *Diagnostic and statistical manual* (4th ed.; text rev.). Washington, DC: Author.

Andreas, C., & Andreas, S. (1989). *Heart of the mind*. Moab, UT: Real People Press.

Argyle, M. (1988*). Bodily communication*, New York: Methuen & Co.

Bailey, A., Le Couteur, A., Gottesman, I., Bolton, P., Simonoff, E., Yuzda, E., & Rutter, M. (1995). Autism as a genetic disorder: Evidence from a British twin study. *Psychological Medicine, 25*, 63-77.

Bandler, R., & Grinder, J. (1979*). Frogs into princes*. Moab, UT: Real People Press.

Barnhill, G., Hagiwara, T., Myles, B. S., & Simpson, R. L. (2000). Asperger Syndrome: A study of the cognitive profiles of 37 children and adolescents. *Focus on Autism and Other Developmental Disabilities, 15*(3), 146-153.

Baron-Cohen S., & Gilberg, C. (1992). Can autism be detected at 18 months? The needle, the haystack, and the CHAT. *British Journal of Psychiatry, 161*, 839.

Baron-Cohen, S. (2000, January). Is Asperger Syndrome/high-functioning autism necessarily a disability? [Invited submission for special millennium issue of *Development and Psychopathology* draft] Cambridge University Press, *12, 269-290.*

Baron-Cohen, S. (2000, January). Is Asperger Syndrome/high-functioning autism necessarily a disability? *Developmental Psychopathology, 12*(3), 489-500.

Baron-Cohen, S. et al. (2000, May). The amygdala theory of autism. *Neuroscience and Behavioral Reviews, 24*(3), 355-364.

Baxter, J. et al. (1992, September). Caudate glucose metabolic rate changes with both drug and behavior therapy for obsessive-compulsive disorder. *Archives of General Psychiatry,* 681-689.

Berthier, M. L., Bayes, A., & Tolosa, E. S. (1993, May). Magnetic resonance imaging in patients with concurrent Tourette's Disorder and Asperger Syndrome. *Journal of the American Academy of Child and Adolescent Psychiatry, 32*(3), 633-639.

Bogdashina, O. (2003). *Different sensory experiences-different sensory worlds*. http://www.autismtoday.com/articles/Different_Sensory_Experiences.htm

Bruun, R. (1994). *A mind of its own.* New York: Oxford University Press.

Burd L., Fisher, W. W., Kerbeshian, J., & Arnold, M. E. (1987). Is the development of Tourette's syndrome a marker for improvement in patients with autism and other developmental disorders? *Journal of the American Academy of Child and Adolescent Psychiatry, 26,* 162-165.

Buron, K. D., & Curtis, M. (2002). *The incredible 5-point scale.* Shawnee Mission, KS: Autism Asperger Publishing Company.

Cederlund, M., & Gilberg, C. (2004, October). One hundred males with Asperger Syndrome: A clinical study of background and associated factors. *Developmental Medicine and Child Neurology, 46*(10), 652-660.

Chang, K. (2004). *Comprehensive treatment of children and adolescents with bipolar disorder.* A workshop syllabus for the Institute for the Advancement of Human Behavior, Portola Valley, CA.

Comings, D. (1991). *Tourette's Syndrome and human behavior.* Duarte, CA: Hope Press.

Comings, D., Freeman, R. D., Fast, D. K., Burd, L., Kerbeshian, J., Robertson, M. M., & Sandor, P. (2000, July). An international perspective on Tourette's syndrome: Selected findings from 3,500 individuals in 22 countries. *Developmental Medicine & Child Neurology, 42,* 436-44.

Critchley, H. D. et al. (2002, November). The functional neuroanatomy of social behavior: Changes in cerebral blood flow when people with autistic disorder process facial expressions. *Brain,* 2203-2212.

DeLong, R. et al. (1994, May). Psychiatric family history and neurological disease in autistic spectrum disorders. *Developmental Medicine and Child Neurology, 36*(5), 441-448.

Duerr, H.A. (Ed.). (2000, November). Comorbid bipolar illness and substance use disorders. Bipolar disorder and impulsive spectrum letter. *Psychiatric Times,* p. 7.

Duran, M. (1998, November). *Tourette's syndrome and obsessive-compulsive behavior.* Presentation at the annual conference of the Washington State Tourette's Syndrome Association, Seattle, WA.

Fletcher, P., Happé, F., Frith, U., Baker, S., Dolan, R., Frackowiak, R., & Frith, C. D. (1995). Other minds in the brain: A functional imaging study of theory of mind in story comprehension. *Cognition, 57*(2), 109-128.

Foa, E. B. et al. (2005). Randomized, placebo-controlled trial of exposure and ritual prevention, clomipramine, and their combination in the treatment of obsessive-compulsive disorder. *American Journal of Psychiatry, 162*(1), 151-161.

Forrest, B. (2004). The utility of math difficulties, internalized psychopathology, and visual-spatial deficits to identify children with the nonverbal learning disability syndrome: Evidence for a visual spatial disability. *Child Neuropsychology, 10*(2), 129-146.

Fox, D. (2002, February). The inner savant (an overview of the work of Dr. Allan Snyder). *Discover, 23*, 2.

Frank, E. (1999, November). Importance of stability in prevention relapse of patients with bipolar disorder. *Journal of Abnormal Psychology, 108*(4), 579-588.

Frazier, J. A., Doyle, R., Chiu, S., & Coyle, J. T. (2002, January). Treating a child with Asperger's Disorder and comorbid bipolar disorder. *American Journal of Psychiatry, 159*, 13-21.

Freeman, R. D., Fast, D. K., Burd, L., Kerbeshian, J., Robertson, M. M., & Sandor P. (2000, July). An international perspective on Tourette's syndrome: Selected findings from 3,500 individuals in 22 countries. *Developmental Medicine & Child Neurology, 42*, 436-444.

Friedlander, L., & Desrocher, M. (2006, January). Neuroimaging studies of obsessive-compulsive disorder in adults and children. *Clinical Psychology Review, 26*(1), 32-49.

Galin, D., & Orstein, R. (1974). Individual differences in cognitive style reflective eye movements. *Neuropsychologia, 12,* 376-397.

Geller, B., & Luby, J. (1997). Child and adolescent bipolar disorder: A review of the past 10 years. *Journal of the American Academy of Child and Adolescent Psychiatry, 36*(9), 1168-1176.

Geller, B., Zimerman, B., Williams, M., Bolhofner, K., Craney, J. L., Delbello, M. P., & Soutullo, C. A. (2000). Diagnostic characteristics of 93 cases of a prepubertal and early adolescent bipolar disorder phenotype by gender, puberty and comorbid attention deficit hyperactivity disorder. *Journal of Child and Adolescent Psychopharmacology, 10*(3), 157-164.

Gilberg, C. (1989). The borderland of autism and Rhett syndrome: Five case histories to highlight diagnostic difficulties. *Journal of Autism and Developmental Disorders, 19*, 545-559.

Glassman, A. H. (1993). Cigarette smoking: Implications for psychiatric illness. *American Journal of Psychiatry, 150*(4), 546-553.

Goldstein, G. et al. (2001). A comparison of WAIS-R profiles in adults with high-functioning autism or differing subtypes of learning disability. *Applied Neuropsychology, 8*(13), 148-154.

Goodwin, F., & Jamison, K. R. (1990*). Manic-depressive illness*. New York: Oxford University Press.

Gracious, B. L., Youngstrom, E. A., Findling, R. L., & Calabrese, J. R. (2002, November). Discriminative validity of a parent version of the Young Mania Rating Scale. *Journal of the American Academy of Child and Adolescent Psychiatry, 41*(11), 1350-1359.

Grandin, T. (1995). *Thinking in pictures and other reports from my life with autism.* New York: Doubleday.

Grandin, T. (2002). *Asperger's and self-esteem: Insight and hope through famous role models.* Arlington, TX: Future Horizons.

Grandin, T. (2005). *My experiences with visual thinking sensory problems and communication difficulties.* Center for the Study of Autism. http://www.autism.org/temple/visual.html

Grandin, T. (2005). *Teaching tips for children and adults with autism.* Center for the Study of Autism. http://www.autism.org/temple/tips.html

Gray, C. (1994). *Comic strip conversations.* Arlington, TX: Future Horizons.

Greene, R. (1998). *The explosive child.* New York: Harper Collins.

Hartmann, T. (1993). *Attention deficit disorder: A different perception.* Grass Valley, CA: Underwood Books.

Hellander, M. (2005). *About pediatric bipolar disorder.* www.http://BDkids.org

Hellander, M. (2005). *Symptoms and accommodations for students with bipolar disorder.* www.http://BDkids.org

Hendren, R. (2004). New research findings in bipolar disorder and pervasive developmental disorder in youth. In *Recent breakthroughs in child and adolescent psychiatry* (pp. 43-70). Irvine, CA: CME Inc.

Hillman, J. (1996). *The soul's code: In search of character and calling.* New York: Random House.

Hindman, J. (1983). *A very touching book.* Baker City, OR: Alexandria Associates.

Hirschfeld, R., Calabrese, J. R., Frye, M. A., Wagner, K. D., & Reed, M. (2003, May). Impact of bipolar depression compared to unipolar depression. *American Psychiatric Association, 4,* 5-13.

Howlin, P., Goode, S., Hutton, J., & Rutter, M. (2004). Adult outcomes in children with autism. *Journal of Child Psychology and Psychiatry, 45*(2), 212-229.

Ishisaka, Y. et al. (1997). Cognitive deficits of autism based on results of three psychological tests. *Japanese Journal of Child and Adolescent Psychiatry, 38*(3), 230-246.

Johnson, K. J., & Layng, T.V.J. (1992). Breaking the structuralist barrier: Literacy and numeracy with fluency. *American Psychologist, 47,* 1475-1490.

Johnson, S. L., Winett, C. A., Meyer, B., & Greenhouse, W. J. (1999, November). Social support and the course of bipolar disorder. *Journal of Abnormal Psychology, 108*(4), 558-567.

Kleinhans, N., Akshoomoff, N., & Delis, D. C. (2005). Executive function in autism and Asperger's disorder: Flexibility, fluency, and inhibition. *Developmental Neuropsychology, 27*(3), 379-401.

Klinkenborg, V. (2005, May). What do animals think? (An interview with Dr. Temple Grandin). *Discover*, 46-52.

Kluth, P. (2005). *A supportive communication partner.* http://www.paulakluth.com

Koppelman, J. (2004, June). Children with mental disorders: Making sense of their needs and the systems that help them. *National Health Policy Forum Issue Brief*, 799.

Kovacs, M., & Pollock, M.S.W. (1995, June). Bipolar disorder and comorbid conduct disorder in children and adolescents. *Journal of the American Academy of Child and Adolescent Psychiatry, 34*(6), 715-723.

Kraepelin, E. (1921). *Manic-depressive paranoia and insanity.* Manchester, NH: Ayer Co Pub. (English translation of the original German from the earlier eighth edition)

Kruesi, M. (2005). Treatment of children with conduct disorder and aggression. In *What's new in child and adolescent psychiatry.* Irving, CA: CME Inc.

Kupka, D. (2003, Fall-Winter). Special report: Rapid cycling vs. non-rapid cycling bipolar disorder. *Bipolar Network News, 9*(2), 4.

Leibenluft, E. (1996, May). Circadian rhythms factor in rapid-cycling bipolar disorder. *Psychiatric Times, 8*, 5.

Losh, M., & Capps, L. (2003, June). Narrative ability in high-functioning children with autism or Asperger Syndrome. *Journal of Autism and Developmental Disorders, 3*, 239-251.

Lynn, G. (1996). *Survival strategies for parenting your ADD child: Dealing with obsessions, compulsions, depression, explosive behavior, and rage.* Grass Valley, CA: Underwood Books.

Lynn, G. (2000). *Survival strategies for parenting children with bipolar disorder.* London, UK: Jessica Kingsley Publishers.

Lynn, J. (2006). *Genius! Nurturing the spirit of the wild, odd, and oppositional child.* London, UK: Jessica Kingsley Publishers.

Maté, G. (1999). *Scattered.* New York: Plume.

Mayes, S. D. (2003). Ability profiles in children with autism: Influence of age and IQ. *Autism, 7*(1), 65-80.

Mayes, S. D. et al. (2004). Similarities and differences in Wechsler Intelligence Scale for Children – Third edition. *Clinical Neuropsychologist, 18*(4), 559-572.

McClure, E., Pope, K., Hoberman, A. J., Pine, D. S., & Leibenluft, E. (2003, June). Facial expression recognition in adolescents with mood and anxiety disorders. *American Journal of Psychiatry, 160,* 1172-1174.

Meade, M. (1993). *Men and the water of life.* San Francisco: Harper.

Mesibov, G. (2000, November-December). High-functioning autism or Asperger Syndrome: Why the controversy? *Autism and Asperger's Digest,* 16-18.

Miklowitz-David, J., & Kim, E. Y. (2002). Childhood mania, attention deficit hyperactivity disorder and conduct disorder; A critical review of diagnostic dilemmas. *Bipolar Disorders, 4*(4), 215-225.

Minshew, N. et al. (1997). Neuropsychologic functioning in autism: Profiles of a complex information processing disorder. *Journal of the International Neuropsychological Society, 3*(4), 303-316.

Muhle, R., Trentacoste, S.V., & Rapin, I. (2004). The genetics of autism. *Pediatrics, 113*(5), 72-86.

*Multidimensional Anxiety Scale for Children.* (1997). Toronto, Canada: Multi-Health Systems.

Myles, B. S. (2001). Using social stories™ and comic strip conversations to interpret social situations for an adolescent with Asperger Syndrome. *Intervention in School and Clinic, 36*(5), 310.

National Institute of Mental Health. (2004, April). *Autism spectrum disorders.* Information Pamphlet, NIH Publication No. 04-5511. http://www.nih.gov

National Institute of Mental Health. (1996 June). Fact Sheet Number PKT 00-0019. *Bipolar disorder.* Prepared with assistance of Hagop Akiskal, Senior Science Advisor, Office of the Director, NIMH.

Nelson, L. (2001). *Communication strategies for adults with autistic spectrum disorders.* http://www.SpeechSense.com

Packer, L. (2005). *OCD awareness exercise for teachers.* http://www.schoolbehavior.com/conditions_ocdawareness.htm

Papolos, D., & Papolos, J. (2000). *The bipolar child.* New York: Broadway Books.

Papolos, D. (2000, January). The hole in the wall gang. *The Bipolar Child Newsletter, 2.* www.bipolarchild.com

Pary, R. J., Levitas, A., & Hurley, A. (1999). Diagnosis of bipolar disorder in persons with developmental disabilities. *Mental Health Aspects of Developmental Disabilities, 2*(2), 37-49.

Perry, W., & Braff, D. L. (1994). Information-processing deficits and thought disorder in schizophrenia. The *American Journal of Psychiatry, 151,* 363-367.

Pfadt, A., Korosh, W., & Wolfson, M. S. (2003, Jan-March). Charting bipolar disorder in people with developmental disabilities. *Mental Health Aspects of Developmental Disabilities, 6*(1), 1-10.

Piaget, J. (1972). *To understand is to invent.* New York: The Viking Press, Inc.

Pickover, C. (1998). *Strange brains: The secret lives of eccentric scientists and madmen.* New York: Harper-Collins.

Popper, C. (1989, Summer). Diagnosing bipolar vs. ADHD. *Journal of the American Academy of Child and Adolescent Psychiatry, 5,* 6.

Post, R. M. (Ed.). (1998, March). Data from the first 200+ patients: Persons diagnosed with BD I, BD II, and BD NOS, show a positive family history rate of 41% for manic-depressive illness. *Bipolar Network News, 4*(1), 1.

Post, R. M. (Ed.). (1999, June). Early recognition and treatment of schizophrenia and bipolar disorder in children and adolescents. Record of presentations, NIMH Research Workshop, Bethesda, MD. *Bipolar Network News, 5*(2), 3.

Prince-Hughes, D. (2004). *Songs of the gorilla nation: My journey through autism.* New York: Harmont Books.

Prigogine, I. (1977). *Self-organization in non-equilibrium systems: From dissipative structures to order through fluctuations.* New York: J. Wiley & Sons.

Purse, M., & Read, K. (2005). *Mary Kay Latourneau, victim of bipolar disorder?* www.about.com

Reilly-Harrington, N. A., Alloy, L. B., Fresco, D. M., & Whitehouse, W. G. (1999, November). Cognitive styles and life events interact to predict bipolar and unipolar symptomology. *Journal of Abnormal Psychology, 108*(4), 567-579.

Reiner, W. G. (2003). Normal and abnormal psychosocial development in children and adolescents. From *Recent breakthroughs in child and adolescent psychiatry* (pp. 13-39). Irvine, CA: CME, Inc.

Rice, J. (1987). The familial transmission of bipolar illness. *Archives of General Psychiatry, 44,* 441-447.

Rinehart, N. J., Bradshaw, J. L., Brereton, A. V., & Tonge, B. J. (2002). Lateralization in individuals with high-functioning autism and Asperger's disorder: A frontostriatal model. *Journal of Autism and Developmental Disorders, 32*(4), 321-331.

Rourke, B. P. (1989). *Nonverbal learning disabilities.* New York: Guilford Press.

Russell, A., Mataix-Cols, D., Anson, M. A., & Murphy, D.G.M. (2005). High prevalence of obsessions and compulsions in Asperger syndrome and high-functioning autism. *British Journal of Psychiatry, 186,* 525-528.

Sabbagh, M. (2004, June). Understanding orbitofrontal contributions to theory-of-mind reasoning: Implications for autism. *Brain and Cognition, 55*(1), 209-215.

Schore, A. (2000, April). Attachment and the regulation of the right brain. *Attachment and Human Development, 2*(1), 23-47.

Sacks, O. (1985). *The man who mistook his wife for a hat.* New York: Summit Books.

Sacks, O. (1995). *An anthropologist on mars.* New York: Knopf.

Sacks, O., with Siebert, E. (1995, May/June). A surgeon's life. *The Family Therapy Networker,* 62-63.

Schreier, H. (2001, September). Socially awkward children: Neurocognitive contributions. *Psychiatric Times, 17,* 9.

Siegel, D. (1999). *The developing mind: How relationships and the brain interact to shape who we are.* New York: Guilford Press.

Silverstein, R. A. (2005). *User's guide to the 2004 IDEA reauthorization.* Consortium for Citizens with Disabilities. www.c-c-d.org

Simoneau, T. L., Miklowitz, D. J., Richards, J. A., Saleem, R., & George, E. L. (1999, November). Bipolar disorder and family communication: Effects of a psychoeducational treatment program. *Journal of Abnormal Psychology, 108*(4), 588.

Strober, M. (1992). Relevance of early age of onset in genetic studies of bipolar affective disorder. *Journal of the American Academy of Child and Adolescent Psychiatry, 31,* 606-610.

Swann, A. (2000, March). *Biology and treatment of impulsivity across and beyond bipolar disorder.* Lecture notes, Stevens Hospital, Edmonds, WA.

The OCD Foundation. (1993). *The touching tree: The story of a child with OCD.* http://ocdfoundation.org

Tsoh, J. Y., Humfleet, G. L., Muñoz, R. F., Reus, V. I., Hartz, D. T., & Hall, S. M. (2000, March). Development of major depression after treatment for smoking cessation. *American Journal of Psychiatry, 157,* 368-374.

Vitiello, M. (1992). Doing it differently. In A. W. Seligman & J. S. Hilkevich, *Don't think about monkeys: Extraordinary stories by people with Tourette's.* Duarte, CA: Hope Press.

Wagner, K. (2004). Diagnosis and treatment of major depression and bipolar disorder in children and adolescents. In *Recent breakthroughs in child and adolescent psychiatry* (pp. 135-162). Irvine, CA: CME, Inc.

Wagner, K. (2005, June). Treatment guidelines for pediatric bipolar disorder. *Psychiatric Times,* 44.

Wilens, T. (1999). *Straight talk about psychiatric medication for kids.* New York: Guilford.

Wilhelm, S., Deckersbach, T., Coffey, B. J., Bohne, A., Alan L. Peterson, A. L., & Baer, L. (2003, June). Habit reversal versus supportive psychotherapy for Tourette's Disorder: A randomized controlled trial. *American Journal of Psychiatry, 160,* 1175-1177.

Williams, D. (1992). *Nobody nowhere – The extraordinary autobiography of an autistic*. New York: Avon Books.

Wing, L. (1981). Asperger Syndrome: A clinical account. *Psychological Medicine, 1*(11), 115-129.

Wing, L. (1993). The definition and prevalence of autism: A review. *European Child and Adolescent Psychiatry, 2*, 1-14.

Young, R. C., Biggs, J. T., Ziegler, V. E., & Meyer, D. A. (1978). A rating scale for mania: Reliability, validity and sensitivity. *British Journal of Psychiatry, 199*, 429-435.

Zinker, J. (1978). *The creative process in gestalt therapy*. New York: Vintage.

# INDEX

## A

ADD. *See* Attention deficit disorder
ADHD. *See* Attention deficit
  hyperactivity disorder
Adolescents
  sports participation, 181
  with AS and BD, 74–75, 76, 85–86
  with bipolar disorder, 38–39
  with high-functioning autism, 188,
    199–200
Adolescents with AS
  gender identity, 29
  sexual issues, 29, 188–189
  teaching methods, 199–200
Alexithymia, 94–95
Anger management, 106–108
Anger triangle, 106–107
Anhedonia, 46
Anxiety
  meltdowns as reaction to, 46
  reducing, 144–148, 153
  relationship to oppositionality,
    140–142
Anxiety disorders, 119, 141, 142
Archetypes
  "Archivist," 97, 111
  "Hermit," 58–59, 97
  "Hunter," 58
  "Scientist," 58–59
  "Warrior," 58–59
"Archivist" archetype, 97, 111
AS. *See* Asperger Syndrome
Asperger, Hans, 17, 18
Asperger-plus diagnoses
  Character Maps, 246–250
  *See also* Bipolar disorder, Asperger
    Syndrome plus; Nonverbal
    learning disability, Asperger
    Syndrome plus; Obsessive
    compulsive disorder, Asperger
    Syndrome plus; Oppositional

defiance disorder, Asperger
  Syndrome plus; Tourette's
  syndrome, Asperger Syndrome
  plus
Asperger Syndrome (AS)
  as stand-alone condition, 17–19
  career success and, 15, 30
  Character Map, 244–245
  creative adults, 26, 260–261
  diagnostic criteria, 16, 18–19,
    163–164, 241–242
  differences from ADD, 233, 234–
    240, 256–257
  differences from HFA, 24–25, 26–
    27, 30–31, 160–163, 164–167,
    168–179, 253
  differences from NLD, 94–97
  differences from Tourette's
    syndrome, 6, 216–222, 255
  differentiation from autism, 18–19
  emergence of symptoms, 19–22,
    25–26
  heritability factors, 15, 28, 50
  myths about, 29
Asperger Syndrome (AS), children
with
  behavioral development, 168–173
  brain differences, 167, 236
  challenges, 9, 17
  cognitive abilities, 19–20
  communication with, 29, 195–197
  creativity, 29, 50, 221
  depression, 49
  educational services, 160–162
  emotional issues, 95, 234–235
  genius, 9–10, 16, 17, 30, 31, 97, 202
  government entitlements, 162
  impairments, 16
  lack of common sense, 20, 49,
    51–52
  math and science performance,
    96–97, 100–101

behaviors at school, 75–76
challenges, 35–36
Character Map, 247
communication with children, 63–65
famous people with, 59
features of neurotype, 49–58
genius, 58–59, 86
in adolescents, 74–75, 76, 85–86
inattention, 51
learning disabilities, 52–53, 79
learning environments, 78–79
mood cycling, 49–50, 60–63
obsessive-compulsive thoughts, 53
positive aspects, 58–59
rage, 51, 53, 65–73
self-care, 52
sexuality, 54
sleep problems, 53
social skills, 51–52
strategies for helping at home, 60–74
strategies for helping at school, 74–85
substance use, 54, 75
suicidality, 55
treatment of BD, 35, 36
Brain
amygdala, 187
cingulate gyrus, 119, 126
dopamine released in playing video games, 146
facial recognition and expression reading, 187
frontal cortex, 25–26
influence of social interaction, 154, 180
lack of communication between right and left hemispheres, 141
left-hemisphere specialization, 25–26, 167
limbic system, 43, 46, 70, 119, 214, 216
orbitofrontal cortex, 25–26, 154

right-hemisphere dysfunction, 91–92, 167
seizures, 45
*See also* Visual thinking
Bullies, 20, 77, 107, 148, 162, 197

# C

Celts, 201–202
Central auditory processing disabilities, 194
Central coherence, weak, 24–25
Character Maps
Asperger-plus clusters, 246–250
Asperger Syndrome, 244–245
criteria, 243
high-functioning autism, 251–253
"look-alike" conditions, 251–257
scoring, 243–244
use of, 258
Child and Adult Bipolar Foundation, 75
Childhood disintegrative disorder, 19
Cigarette smoking, 54, 75
Cognitive abilities, 19–20
Community responsibility, building sense of, 180–185
Compulsions
distinction from special interests, 117–118
in AS children, 115–116, 117, 118–119, 121–123
in AS plus BD, 53
in Tourette's syndrome, 214, 215–216
natural response prevention, 125–126
*See also* Obsessive compulsive disorder
Computers
classroom use, 200
hand-held, 111
interest in, 31
software writing skills, 174
Coprolalia, 213, 214

Counterwill, 143, 144–148, 153
Creativity
  of adults with AS, 26, 260–261
  of children with AS, 29, 50, 221
  of children with Tourette's
    syndrome, 219, 221
Cyclothymic disorder, 36

# D

Darwin, Charles, 120
Depression
  definition, 37
  in children with AS, 49
  physical features, 37
  *See also* Bipolar disorder
Diagnoses
  complexity, 5–7
  criteria for Asperger Syndrome, 16,
    18–19, 163–164, 241–242
  identifying trunk neurotype, 215
  seeing child's spirit through,
    259–260
  *See also* Character Maps
*Diagnostic and Statistical Manual*
  (DSM-IV), 16, 18, 35, 51, 163–164,
  215, 233–234
Dopamine, 146
Drugs. *See* Medications
DSM-IV. *See Diagnostic and
  Statistical Manual*

# E

Edison, Thomas, 59, 260
Education. *See* Schools
Einstein, Albert, 10
Emotions
  alexithymia, 94–95
  awareness and labeling, 106–107
  lack of theory of mind, 141–142
  of AS children, 95, 234–235
  of AS plus NLD children, 99
  understanding others', 187–188, 235

Encephalopathy not otherwise
  specified, 36
Executive function, 19–20, 52, 234
Eye movements, 173–174, 175

# F

Families
  building relationships with AS-
    plus-ODD children, 148–153
  parenting strategies, 162–163,
    179–189
  routines, 144–145, 180
  strategies for helping AS-plus-BD
    children, 60–74
  strategies for helping AS-plus-
    OCD children, 124–130
  strategies for helping AS-plus-
    ODD children, 144–147
  *See also* Heritability factors
FBA. *See* Functional behavior
  assessment
Fight-or-flight behavior, 38–39, 43,
  92, 217–218
Figures of speech, 21–22, 189, 198
Fixed-figure perceptual style, 22–24,
  25–27, 147, 164–166
Friends, 217, 236
  *See also* Social skills
Full-field perceptual style, 24–25,
  26–27, 164–166
Functional behavior assessment
  (FBA), 81

# G

GAD. *See* Generalized anxiety
  disorder
GCBF. *See* Georgia Child Bipolar
  Foundation
Gender identity, 29, 188
Generalized anxiety disorder (GAD),
  141, 142
Genetic factors. *See* Heritability factors